# Feel

# Younger

## How to Improve Your Strength, Mobility Energy and Vitality to Feel Younger

*(Practically Proven Steps to Look, Feel and Act Younger Even as You Age)*

**Charlie Wilson**

Published By **Ryan Princeton**

# Charlie Wilson

*Feel Younger: How to Improve Your Strength, Mobility Energy and Vitality to Feel Younger (Practically Proven Steps to Look, Feel and Act Younger Even as You Age)*

ISBN   978-1-998901-33-3

Legal & Disclaimer

## TABLE OF CONTENTS

# Chapter 1: The Science Behind Red Light Therapy And Why It's Miles Good For Us

Red mild remedy is a in particular new restoration method that uses low levels of pink wavelengths of moderate to deal with one-of-a-kind pores and pores and skin issues. The pores and pores and skin troubles that can be dealt with are: Wrinkles, scars, and continual wounds, to name some. Back within the early Nineties, purple moderate remedy turn out to be furthermore used by a few scientists to help increase vegetation at the equal time as they were in location. Scientists positioned that there may be an immoderate mild that is emitted from the crimson slight emitting diodes that allows to promote increase and the photosynthesis method in plant cells. Red light remedy turned into moreover studied to appearance if it is able to be utilized in packages of medicine. Researchers desired to look if it become feasible for crimson moderate treatment to boom the power indoors human cells. They believed that if it emerge as feasible, it might be an effective manner to cope with muscle atrophy, slow wound restoration, and assist deal with bone-density problems that astronauts are plagued with because of the weightlessness they revel in on the equal time as on location journey expeditions.

Red moderate treatment has been round for a long time, and it has been known through many one-of-a-kind names. You may additionally have heard of purple slight remedy earlier than, and in reality did now not understand it. Red mild treatment is likewise referred to as the subsequent:
• Soft laser treatment
• Cold laser remedy
• Photonic stimulation
• Biostimulation

- Low-diploma mild remedy (LLLT)
- Photobiomodulation (PBM)
- Low-strength laser treatment (LPLT)

Red mild remedy also can be applied in brilliant types of drug remedies in which the pink light is used to photosensitize the medicine. This is commonly referred to as "photodynamic remedy". The mild will extremely good feature an activating agent for the medicine. Red mild beds are normally decided in salons, as it's miles stated to help with reducing splendor pores and skin troubles like stretch marks and wrinkles. It can also be applied in maximum clinical medical institution settings to treat extra severe scientific conditions collectively with psoriasis, slow-healing wounds, or maybe the side outcomes which might be associated with chemotherapy. There is lots of evidence that it's miles a promising remedy for certain pores and skin conditions.

How it Works

One gain of purple slight remedy is its potential to work via producing biochemical results inside the cells of the body that allows to boost the inherent mitochondria. The mitochondria is in which the cell's electricity is created, for this reason making it the powerhouse of the mobile. The molecule that is determined in all cells of dwelling subjects is the energy-wearing cells referred to as the "adenosine triphosphate" (ATP). Using crimson mild therapy to growth the feature of the mitochondria lets in the mobile to make extra of the ATP. When cells have extra electricity, it turns into less tough for them to function extra successfully, rejuvenate themselves at a faster fee, and restore damage greater speedy. Red slight remedy differs from laser and intense pulsed slight (IPL) treatment alternatives because of the truth crimson mild remedy does no longer reason harm to the floor of the pores and pores and skin. Laser and pulsed slight treatment alternatives are mentioned to paintings by the use of developing a managed location of harm to the outer most layer of the pores and pores and skin, so you can bring about the begin of tissue repair. Red mild therapy is capable of bypass round this harsh pores and pores and pores and skin damage via using straight away going to the step of stimulating the regeneration of new pores and pores and pores and skin. The moderate that is emitted from crimson slight treatment is able to move extra or much less 5 millimeters beneath the pores and pores and pores and skin's ground. Therefore, it does no longer need to create harm at the outermost layer of the pores and pores and pores and skin.

Red mild has a deep-tissue penetration that isn't always to be had through one-of-a-type coloured lighting fixtures. This manner that pink moderate ought to have a systemic effect at the frame of a human, in place of the organic outcomes of the purple mild last only in the localized vicinity in which it's miles performed. The systemic effects are from pink mild remedy's potential to stimulate ATP manufacturing. The devices which is probably carried out in purple mild remedy may be made in a way that lets in them to emit very particular moderate wavelengths. The complete goal of the red moderate treatment devices is to have an effect on the mitochondria at some point of all of the frame. Improving the overall function of the mitochondria will beautify the general health of your body. Not all of the pink mild wavelengths and infrared lights are absorbed in maximum beneficial degrees within the mitochondria. By the usage of purple mild remedy to reason the mild-emitting diodes (LEDs) within the course of the just a few restoration wavelengths it is able to absorb, you are then probably to carry out the maximum quantity of absorption,thereby getting the extraordinary effects.

The Benefits of Red Light Therapy to Health and Wellness

The Food and Drug Administration (FDA) has criminal red moderate treatment as a steady and powerful treatment for medicinal functions. Scientists have created lots of studies on crimson light remedy through the years, which incorporates medical trials that have been peer-reviewed, and lots of also are posted in maximum crucial clinical journals. There is masses of overwhelming evidence in select of the effectiveness and protection of crimson moderate remedy. In truth, crimson slight remedy has been felony with the aid of the FDA as a manner to heal joint pain and non-life threatening conditions like wrinkle reduce price. It is concept to be a more stable opportunity to drug treatments and surgical tactics, and lots of humans are leaning in the direction of red slight treatment over traditional remedies because of the truth it's far rather cheaper. It also does now not deliver the danger of life-threatening troubles that are frequently concerned with surgical strategies, and tablets that may have horrible issue outcomes.

Anti-Aging Benefits

Red mild treatment advocates and clients have referred to that there can be a feeling of rejuvenation after its use. The reason for that is that it stimulates the introduction of collagen. When collagen is produced, it aids the strengthening of your hair. Moreover, it makes your pores and skin extra elastic, and your connective tissues enhance its feature of maintaining the whole lot collectively. Several studies have located out that red moderate treatment allows revitalize complexion and skin tone. It furthermore moderates out of doors growing antique symptoms and signs and allows accelerate the recovery time associated with wounding and scarring. Many celebrities have taken to pink moderate remedy and often visit spas and moreover use at domestic treatment plans with the intention to experience the pores and skin advantages of red mild treatment.

## Muscle Growth and Recovery

Red moderate remedy is now being utilized by athletes and elite trainers to assist enhance muscle increase and acquire the advantages of muscle recovery. It has been cited and debated if pink mild treatment may be an unfair gain in a few aggressive sports activities activities, regardless of it being truely natural! NFL stars and UFC warring parties also are appeared for talking publicly approximately using pink light remedy to get higher after annoying sporting sports. Studies and trials have proven that it lets in your frame to generate a first rate quantity of cellular power and reduce oxidative stress, and this helps tissue repair, thereby assisting worn-out and damaged muscle mass get better.

Moreover, it allows regenerate new tissues extra speedy. In a take a look at done in 2016, it come to be positioned that the use of red slight treatment additionally bolsters the development of wholesome muscle companies, which now not extremely good increases energy, but additionally muscle length and bulk as properly. Red slight treatment isn't always only seemed for muscle recovery, however furthermore stepped forward intercourse stress and testosterone production. Many top non-public going for walks shoes swear with the aid of manner of it. Those who're struggling with their intercourse drives declare that red mild treatment is a herbal way for them to increase it without garnering any risky difficulty effects.

Inflammation and Joint Pain

One fine effect this is most typically said in crimson slight treatment is that it promotes a reduction in infection and oxidative strain, which allows many customers of crimson light treatment reduce their joint ache. Many individuals who be stricken by chronic ache, which includes the factor effect of fibromyalgia, and want to reduce their infection, have recommended that their pain stages had been extensively decreased after the usage of purple mild remedy. Using this could be precise for people who experienced an increase in infection because of accidents. It moreover facilitates patients who're older and who experience more joint ache as they age. Many people become having surgical tactics because of the reality their joint pain and infection have no longer been well addressed and treated. Red mild remedy will useful resource in reducing the massive kind of lifelong issues humans can experience, further to limit the amount of surgeries people could in all likelihood need due to contamination and joint pain.

Melatonin and Sleep
In this point in time, many people are exposed to horrific artificial slight for loads hours within the daylight. When we come

domestic, we reveal ourselves to the blue mild of our TVs, computer structures, and clever gadgets. Artificial slight is bad because it disrupts our circadian rhythm, making it hard for us to go to sleep without a doubt. On the alternative, crimson moderate remedy aids in the safety of our internal body clock from being tormented by the synthetic moderate that surrounds us continuously. Studies have tested that red slight treatment moreover will growth the herbal manufacturing of melatonin, it is a chemical that permits the frame nod off and is simply produced in our our bodies. Many people suffer from a lack of melatonin, and regularly take synthetic nutritional supplements to help them fall asleep. Red mild therapy is a greater herbal way for humans to boom melatonin production, and assist them doze off quicker and be capable of experience more restful sleep at night time time time.

Increase in Thyroid Function and Fat Loss

Red slight remedy is understood for growing the hormones produced by means of your thyroids. These hormones are very critical because of the reality they are the hormones answerable for ok energy manufacturing within the human frame. The thyroid is the most crucial variable accountable for energy manufacturing in the frame. It is one of the most crucial factors of the frame as it creates energy degrees which might be immoderate sufficient so that you will now not feel gradual. Red slight treatment can assist decorate signs and symptoms and situations of hypothyroidism. Red mild remedy ought to be accomplished to the thyroid on the body for extended intervals of time. It is examined that a measurable difference inside the feature of the thyroid can be completed inside each week of utilizing pink mild remedy to the location every day.

Sunburn Damage Prevention and Treatment

There is likewise proof that you may use red light remedy to help save you sunburns or decrease the intensity of sunburn. To save you sunburns, you could use purple slight remedy for a couple of minutes earlier than stepping out into direct sunlight hours. Red light remedy is belief to protect you from sunburns due to the reality the infrared mild is in reality saved for your frame. The morning sun also consists of excessive quantities of infrared moderate. Red moderate therapy permit you to prevent sunburns later in the day if you are exposed to daylight hours for an prolonged time frame. To use it to get over sunburns, exercise pink moderate remedy at the affected areas for just a few minutes. Red moderate treatment is proper for assisting decorate pores and skin restoration in situations of immoderate pressure (like sunburn). Red mild remedy additionally helps you produce more melanin, just so your pores and skin can be less possibly to have terrible reactions even as out inside the sun due to the fact you'll be used to the exposure through the crimson slight treatment.

Oral Health Improvement

Red moderate remedy can be used for oral care as properly. Applied at once to tooth, crimson light treatment can decrease the tiers of hypersensitivity some human beings revel in of their enamel. This approach that human beings will not have a horrible response after they devour or drink some thing heat or cold, depending at the sensitivity level of their teeth. Red mild treatment is also appeared to lessen the extent of dangerous mouth micro organism that could reason infections of the mouth, and it additionally heals wounds within the gums so that you do now not get exposed to bacteria that would doubtlessly get into the accidents and reason infections. Our mouth is the location of our our our bodies the has the most germs, so decreasing the volume of bacteria in our mouth in a steady way will

15

now not handiest advantage our tooth and gums, but can even assist prevent us from getting unwell extra often. Red mild treatment is likewise used for the recovery of enamel bone after a teeth has professional some harm.

Hair Loss Reversal

Red slight remedy is thought for its capability to opposite hair loss in every women and men. Red mild remedy has end up a most appropriate desire in comparison to pharmaceuticals which might be typically used to opposite hair loss. The purpose for that is that maximum prescribed drugs consist of risky issue effects that many humans would love to avoid. While crimson light treatment is not an ordinary solution for hair loss—this means that, no longer absolutely everyone can also have incredible consequences from using red moderate treatment for hair loss—but such things as prescribed drugs aren't installation, both. Red light remedy is a more non-invasive technique to hair loss, and it's miles more commonly used to address hair loss than different styles of invasive tactics. Personally, I may additionally an lousy lot as an alternative attempt red mild remedy for hair loss over taking a tablet that might not artwork, and then having to deal with the functionality thing outcomes which can be frequently related to taking prescription medicine.

Pain Tolerance

Red mild remedy is understood to be effective in decreasing pain that is related to situations which includes osteoarthritis, again ache, and precise joint problems. Red mild therapy is likewise a viable treatment for migraine complications on the same time because the crimson slight is done right now to the pinnacle. This is wonderful for people who suffer from commonplace complications and do not pick out possibility treatment inside the market. Those drugs in the market for migraines have horrible facet consequences, and those emerge as in worse conditions after taking them, and but they despite the fact that enjoy headaches often. With all the research this is available on the use of pink light remedy for treating exquisite ranges of ache, pink mild therapy indicates promise in treating brilliant stages of ache in various elements of the body.

Mood Changes
When pink light is implemented to the top and skull, it may penetrate deep down into the brain. Applying the mild in your brain only a few minutes an afternoon has shown to decrease the results of anxiety and despair. While it isn't confirmed for this shape of treatment to have any factor outcomes associated with them, it's miles advocated that you talk to a medical doctor and do your private studies earlier than performing this form of remedy on your very personal. The nice possibility for this sort of treatment is to shop for a device that is preconfigured from the software program to the thoughts as it

would automatically recognize the stages of mild to apply and the way prolonged you must be exposed to it. This manner, you could guarantee your self which you are receiving the advanced degree of remedy, and you are not inflicting any capability harm for your mind, as red mild treatment is not usually carried out to this vicinity of the body. Many people who've been using purple slight treatment for precise kinds of treatment have additionally seen their moods appreciably beautify at the equal time as they maintain to do the remedy. It can be that the remedy is responsible for the development, or that it's far honestly treating the location in which it's miles used, after which the customers experience more awesome because of the truth they no longer enjoy the equal terrible symptoms they used to have in advance than they commenced the pink mild treatment.

Safe, Non-Invasive, and Drug-Free

Unlike pretty some the traditional treatments which might be used for the problems we indexed above, purple mild remedy is steady, does now not require invasive technology, and is sincerely unfastened of medicine. Red mild remedy moreover does now not have any terrible element outcomes which may be regularly associated with one in all a type sorts of treatments. It is one of the maximum innocent herbal restoration therapies. This precise sort of mild brings targeted power that has a better score in assessment to the solar but with out the dangerous effect of UV rays that might have a protracted-lasting impact. People round the place are seeing the rejuvenating benefits of purple light treatment in their ordinary recoveries, and it's miles one of the most sought-after technology within the marketplace because it has the least quantity of dangerous results that comparable era have. Many crimson light treatment devices use pretty green and medicinal-grade LEDs which is probably, via a top notch deal, the superb manner to bring about the right mild depth and wavelengths which may be applied in red moderate remedy. These LEDs are critical in complete body slight remedy. LEDs are able to produce the precise wavelength of slight this is carried out at a incredible performance minus the warmth generated from their use. LEDs are stated to remaining 25 instances longer at least, in contrast to incandescent bulbs. In addition, they will be not as delicate and are a good deal lots much less probable to interrupt. LEDS have been recognized to be a revolutionizing strain in lights during the last many years, and that they have made it possible for us to use effective and solid mild treatment inside the consolation of our very non-public houses. Moreover, many humans can be able to have sufficient cash it due to the fact its fee is possible for maximum human beings.

LED Red Light

Unlike older fashion lights like incandescent bulbs, LEDs are designed inside the shape of manner that they might best emit a light that is preprogrammed very particularly for restoration wavelengths of light. Being capable of emit at a restoration wavelength makes LED bulbs maximum beneficial for red slight treatment. It is presently not viable for bulbs that aren't LEDs to pinnacle on the precise wavelengths needed to be considered at a restoration level. Halogen bulbs, further to the incandescent, emit non-forestall spectrums of slight. This continuous light spectrum isn't always actual for maximizing the healing benefits of mild, specifically in pink moderate remedy. You will really need bulbs which can be LED and feature very precise healing output stages which includes 620mn, 660nm, and 810nm, relying at the shape of remedy you need to get maintain of. Red mild treatment options typically use each red and infrared wavelengths. These wavelengths are used because of their capability to penetrate very deeply into the tissues of the body. They also are with out troubles absorbable in the frame for handiest benefits to be administered.

As we've now found out, moderate does no longer simplest function as seen shades that let you see your surroundings, however it's miles certainly penetrating into your frame. It in the end has organic effects inside the body, much like photosynthesis and the results that mild has on vegetation. If you take a look at photos of mild and the manner it's far absorbed in the body, you may be capable of see that pink moderate has a greater penetration degree as compared to fantastic kinds of mild. This way that pink slight can acquire deeper tiers of frame tissues than specific types of mild, and for that reason we're capable of see the most blessings from the red mild treatment. Other wavelengths of light can not acquire deep within the tissues and consequently, have no effect at the underlying issues in a way that pink mild remedy is known to do. Not all red slight and infrared wavelengths are optimally absorbed thru the mitochondria in the body, however. By focused on the LEDs toward the few restoration wavelengths, you are much more likely to carry out most absorption. In cross decrease returned, if you are not the usage of wavelengths which might be pleasant, their electricity is maximum probably wasted. Traditional bulbs use an entire lot of those middleman wavelengths that do not have any tested recovery outcomes at the body because of the fact there isn't always enough mild emitted on the wavelength peaks which might be desired for therapeutic ranges.

## Chapter 2: Weight Loss With Red Light Therapy

Losing weight and fats loss are in all likelihood the most often talked about topics amongst human beings in masses of societies. People want to shed pounds and fat for each scientific and beauty motives. Some people may also additionally need to shed kilos for health reasons, as it might in all likelihood lessen the signs and symptoms and signs which may be proper away related to being obese and moreover help them enjoy better. Being overweight may be some element that takes location because of overeating or an unregulated weight loss program. It additionally can be a detail effect of each different contamination and drugs taken to deal with extraordinary clinical troubles. Some people need to shed pounds because of the reality they recognize they will look better in their clothes and enjoy greater assured of their relationships and careers.

It isn't unexpected that masses of human beings revel in that they are no longer wherein they want to be of their jobs or relationships due to the fact they may be overweight. Regardless of the reasons in the returned of the desires of weight loss, people are searching out more secure alternatives to weight reduction, capsules, and shakes. These have been as soon as wildly popular, but with wholesome food and natural eating turning into more well-known, people are sincerely searching for to shift from the artificial weight reduction regime that makes use of drug treatments to extra non-invasive weight loss techniques. Red moderate treatment is an up-and-coming approach to weight reduction, and as we already apprehend, it is a non-invasive method of having effects that humans want.

We already recognize what crimson mild remedy can do for our cells. Research research have decided that crimson mild treatment not simplest permits our body

26

energize itself a long way greater efficaciously, however moreover affects adiposities, which can be the cells in which the body stores fats and brings the lipids to scatter. In first-rate terms, this way has the capability to useful resource the frame to cleanse the cells of saved fats actually. It will increase the strength produced in cells, and they work greater hard than ever to help electricity production.Therefore, the frame will rely upon the cells wherein fats is saved to preserve its diploma of strength. When the frame begins to depend upon the fat cells for power, the fat manifestly gets burned off effectively, and a common detail impact of that is weight reduction that can be visible visibly from outside of the frame. Red mild remedy lets in those who want to shed pounds keep a wholesome life-style with out the want to starve themselves. We all recognise that when we circulate hunger mode, our our our our bodies simply keep onto the fat cells in our bodies so that you can live alive. Light remedy has wonderful abilties that would affect the way the body sheds fat and weight. Red moderate treatment can have an effect on starvation degrees, that can assist someone who is liable to overeating cast off the accumulation of extra fat storage earlier than it's far saved. Red mild remedy is verified in studies to assist manipulate immoderate stages of hormones, along side ghrelin and leptin, that have an impact on the sensation of hunger that sufferers who are regularly disadvantaged of sleep tend to enjoy.

Clinical research has hooked up that purple slight therapy enables reduce fats and aids people with weight control. One scientific studies suggests that pink moderate remedy had been instrumental to supporting in cellulite loss among members of different age stages and body types; therefore, it's miles said to have the capacity to control weight troubles. In terms of physical look, it allows beauty body enhancement with its many amazing consequences on fat discount. A lot of human beings are turning a ways from the traditional forms of weight reduction and as an opportunity accepting the generation of near infrared and pink mild treatment options as they'll be non-invasive, natural, and harmless alternatives to amazing weight reduction strategies. It helped them emerge as extra healthful and extra wholesome than they were in comparison to operating on it on their private. Most of the time, the outcomes that human beings see from the crimson light treatment moreover allowed them to alternate their way of lifestyles behavior which can have been maintaining them from looking and feeling the manner they need to. The pink mild therapy does no longer best provide fantastic bodily effects, however furthermore assist them exercise greater and eat greater healthy with a purpose to keep their effects. This lets in them to vicinity their remedy to accurate use. Humans truely start to art work greater tough once they see outcomes, and starting with pink moderate treatment is a high-quality step to stay a higher and more healthy lifestyle. However, they can't constantly hit the ground taking walks without some steering and seeing effects in different approaches first. There are many extraordinary health blessings on health and weight reduction which have been decided with the system of crimson moderate remedy, and we are happy to speak approximately the special tiers of weight loss that people will experience once they begin using red mild treatment for this purpose.

Studies Regarding Cellulite

There became a have a have a look at finished in 2011 that end up approximately purple moderate therapy and its effect on cellulite cut price. Women most of the a long time of 25 and fifty five were damaged up into super companies for this look at. Women within the first institution used pink moderate remedy and did a few shape of a treadmill workout alongside aspect their remedies. The ladies within the second group did now not accumulate the purple mild therapy, however further they did a few form of treadmill exercise. The take a look at come to be carried out in a series of weeks just so the exercising and purple mild remedy might also supply effects based on what the ladies have been receiving: Just the exercise or each the purple moderate remedy and the exercise. The researchers then took thermographic images of all the members to peer the variations the numerous two organizations. The photographs indicated that the adjustments in their thigh circumference, in addition to the amount of cellulite that girls had on their thighs, have grow to be considerably decreased with the pink moderate treatment and exercising mixed. The women who truly did treadmill bodily games decreased their cellulite however not as loads as the first corporation of women did. This examine modified into succesful to expose that treadmill exercise with crimson mild remedy periods art work together to enhance body aesthetic more so than ladies who honestly begin through exercise. Red moderate remedy may be the jumpstart to fat loss and cellulite cut price that you need that permits you to maintain pushing yourself to change your manner of lifestyles for the better. Red light treatment is proper for your arrogance due to the truth lowering your cellulite will probably make you sense snug in your private body. You can start to construct yourself-self assure, especially even as you are out on the beach, or you may put on outfits that you otherwise couldn't put on because of the fact you are not confident in conjunction with your pores and pores and pores and skin and body.

Cosmetic Contouring of the Body
Most people need to lose weight to appearance higher once they see themselves within the reflect or after they

recognize that they may be going to the seashore and need to rock their bathing in form. Most people try quick fixes and get discouraged due to the reality they may be now not seeing the effects that they want, or they see results right away, however no longer outcomes that could stick spherical. These forms of fixes aren't accurate in your shallowness or your fitness. Now, it is turning into more common for people to look tons much less invasive alternations which may be higher for his or her our our bodies. There are many forms of remedies that concentrate on fat and enhance look, and you may have heard of them being known as "frame contouring" or "frame sculpting". Some of these frame contouring and frame sculpting remedy options are surgical, and a few are non-invasive. These are some of the primary spa-kind recuperation tactics which have made people become interested in non-invasive fat loss technology. However, plenty of the ones kinds of treatments are appeared to artwork plenty much less successfully. Sometimes, they're powerful however would probable take such numerous intervals in advance than consequences may be visible. As a cease end end result, many ladies become spending loads of greenbacks on treatment options that are not as powerful or does not closing once they may be stopped. Oftentimes, those forms of treatment plans moreover have horrible and bothersome aspect outcomes. The proper treatment, but, must were tested and examined in improving your frame's contour. They need to be non-invasive and really herbal in all its office work. It additionally should make you sense great, especially at the same time as you look in the replicate or try on bathing fits on your beach tour. There are many benefits to looking and feeling true in your non-public body, and pink mild remedy has allowed girls to peer the results they may be looking for in an cheaper manner in which they do no longer need to worry about feeling the horrible element consequences. The most effective aspect results of red mild generation are the very outcomes that they may be looking for.

Experience Less Girth and a Smaller Waistline

Women have troubles about their waistline and the numerous things that they may do to hold a smaller waistline. Waist jogging footwear have been exceptionally well-known within the past years but have fallen off the marketplace due to the fact many human beings have determined out how terrible it became for his or her frame. It ought to without a doubt crush your ribs and inner organs. We aren't within the day and age in which corsets are a want to appear adorable, and we should all prevent subjecting ourselves to this kind of torture simply to appearance lovely for society's requirements. There were research accomplished in double-blind conditions wherein purple light remedy changed into used on individuals at 635 - 800 nanometers in a span of 4 weeks. A double-blind have a observe is on the identical time as every the people and the researchers do not understand which people inside the corporations are truely receiving the remedy and people who're receiving a placebo. A "placebo" is a few aspect this is utilized in a study as a control to replace the product that is being studied. The purple moderate remedy modified into applied directly to the waistline of a number of the members; others were given the placebo. After the four-week time period, they recorded the effects of the treatment on the dimensions of their waistlines. The splendid consequences have been in select of the pink mild remedy: The ladies who had obtained the real remedy had a substantial reduction in their waistline girth in desire to folks who had only gotten the placebo.

Targeted Fat Loss

Red mild remedy may be used for targeting fats loss in superb places of the body. Many human beings have pain points of their body and this influences their outward appearance, however a few humans may not always need to paintings on their entire body or look. There are not many remedies handy for fats loss that assist you to purpose advantageous areas of the frame. Many of those are invasive treatments, i.E., those inside the shape of tablets that requires the product to go into into the body and bloodstream so as for it to art work, thereby affecting the entire frame. Studies have examined that the use of pink moderate treatment allows customers experience a good sized decrease in elegant fats in the place in which they finished pink slight remedy, and it could be used in hundreds of virtually one in all a type factors of the body as well. This is incredible for human beings who've undesirable fat in locations in which it's far difficult to use a exercise, and the pink slight remedy allows them to intention the ones regions mainly on the manner to get maintain of better effects. The duration of particular frame regions wherein the purple mild treatment modified into used become reduced, and this resulted inside the outward appearance that humans had been aiming for. Red slight remedy is natural, so it's miles possible to apply it to multiple intricate regions of the body so long as you are the usage of an appropriate wavelength and publicity times. You can also consult a medical doctor who specializes in crimson mild remedy to understand what ought to paintings wonderful for your areas of situation, and you could moreover follow what you positioned at domestic if you decide that home remedy is what you want, whilst you start the use of pink mild treatment. Targeted regions might also embody: Your hands, legs, and butt.

Tighten Your Hips and Thighs

As stated above, girls inside the past regularly grew to become to weight running footwear to lessen the circumference in their waist and hips on the way to benefit a look that curvy ladies with smaller waist have. Studies have determined that this kind of contortion isn't always right for our frame and our fitness, so they're attempting to find strategies which is probably a good buy much less painful. In the improvement of laser treatment, some research confirmed that there are benefits from red slight remedy whilst used at 635nm to apply contouring on areas which incorporates the hips, thighs, and waist. By the stop of the take a look at that turn out to be carried out for the scale good deal of hips and thighs, the mean lack of fats must be almost 3 inches inside the regular duration of the place. These areas, mainly, noticed a notable good buy in duration whilst the treatment come to be used at this wavelength for this meant reason. It is confirmed that this wavelength and device is solid to apply on the ones areas of the frame, and it served its reason of decreasing the dimensions of thighs and hips. Since the ones are hassle areas for max women, the purple moderate remedy is most commonly applied on them, and women do no longer want to fear about causing harm to the organs which can be near the ones regions in their our bodies. Researches have studied how red moderate remedy can affect the ones regions of the frame, and have been in a position to show that it is stable and clinically powerful to be used within the reduce charge of the scale of hips and thighs. Using crimson slight remedy together with a physical exercise will in reality allow the consumer to appearance appropriate consequences, because of the reality the purple mild remedy will jumpstart one's development. In addition, walking out will help maintain the right duration of one's waist and thighs and reason them to enterprise whilst they lose fat.

Weight Control and Obesity

In 2015, some Brazilian researchers piloted a take a look at that evaluated the consequences of every bodily exercise and purple mild therapy. The have a look at's individuals have been sixty 4 girls a number of the some time of 20 and 40 years vintage, and who had been considered obese. Obese girls on this age group greater frequently have problems dropping weight because their hormones frequently exchange, and as a end result, so do their life. It furthermore is predicated upon on in the event that they have got youngsters and if they're in relationships. Women's our bodies commonly have a tendency to alternate substantially at this age variety, and that they normally discover it more difficult to shed pounds. In addition, they'll fail to have the motivation and strength to workout to maintain weight loss and appearance and experience real about themselves. Sometimes, exercising isn't the great difficulty that girls want so as to reduce their stage of weight problems, and they often achieve within the path of greater invasive strategies to look desired effects brief. When they do, they do no longer see that the outcomes closing lengthy. In the have a have a observe, one employer finished carrying sports activities and received particular levels of treatment regarding purple light treatment . The manage institution, alternatively, achieved physical video games with out receiving any treatment on crimson mild remedy. The researchers had been in a function to complete that after seeking out to reduce the mass of fat in the female frame, the purple slight treatment,even as carried out with an workout routine, modified into more powerful than exercising by myself. They have been additionally able to determine that the purple slight remedy, at the thing of an exercising regular, furthermore accelerated skeletal muscle agencies. This manner that crimson moderate treatment can assist enhance the blessings of bodily exercising in obese women as it lets in promote tremendous adjustments in in any other case inflexible metabolic profiles. This manner that it has helped enhance the metabolism of these obese girls and helped them shed pounds to gain their lives and produce their fitness again into suitable tiers. A modern-day check turn out to be additionally achieved on more youthful ladies who have been considered to be obese, and that they confirmed similar outcomes much like the Brazilian study of the girls who've been taken into consideration center aged. The more youthful girls in the 2nd examine confirmed that workout and crimson moderate treatment finished together had better results than the girls who just exercised.

A critical advantage of crimson moderate remedy is that you can do the remedies your self at home. This manner that you could deliver your self quick treatment times without having to go to the health practitioner's place of job, and you're regardless of the fact that capable of see the equal consequences. This keeps girls endorsed to keep remedy as they could no longer have an excuse no longer to get the treatments if they will be some distance from their home. In addition, they do not have to expose their our our bodies in public till they revel in more assured of their new our bodies which have benefited from the pink slight remedy. This manner, they will customise the way they accumulate red moderate remedy treatments at domestic to make sure that they are using the correct wavelength and exposure instances which is probably precise to their frame and the form of treatment they want to get maintain of. This permits them to experience absolutely snug of their treatments, and they do no longer need to fear about awesome humans judging them for receiving the treatment.

Moreover, you may see your very very own outcomes in real time whilst not having to depend upon someone to can help you realize what works and what doesn't. It can be a battle for ladies who realise what they want, but as an opportunity need to combat with professionals an super way to get the varieties of remedy they want and deserve. Doing it yourself lets in you the gain of doing the remedies to your personal time table – as we're all busy with our lives and can't continuously make it to a health practitioner's workplace, specifically while scientific medical doctors might not have on hand administrative center hours that suits us.

In summary, medical research has confirmed that pink mild remedy is one of the terrific non-invasive technology in terms of supporting ladies lose weight whilst they're now not getting the effects they may be expecting through workout by myself. Red moderate remedy is a examined herbal remedy that is solid and effective, especially on fat loss and weight control. It is likewise a excellent approach of splendor development that works on targeted regions for body contouring. Whether you want to shed pounds for fitness motives or for splendor motives, pink moderate remedy works for each and is one of the nice within the marketplace. More importantly, purple light treatment does no longer offer you with any undesirable thing results. This allows you to do the remedy and keep about your existence and day without any downtime or awful results on your body, in that you may emerge as worse off than you were in advance than administering the remedy. If you revel in that you want to test out the medical journals which have been posted about the great consequences of purple slight remedy on weight reduction, you need to enjoy unfastened to search around the net for credible scientific journals, and notice them for yourself! This e-book is a guide as a way to discern out if pink moderate remedy is right for you, however it is also vital that you are looking for recommendation from medical specialists to make sure that your clinical statistics could probable permit you to see the benefits of crimson slight remedy. Red slight remedy is the amazing non-invasive remedy to be had for weight loss, and it has actually taken off inside the weight loss market, specifically now that human beings are refusing to apply tablets and shakes that could rather have adverse results on the body and standard health.

# Chapter 3: Addressing Safety Concerns And Skin Issues

As with all new treatments within the market, there is mostly a state of affairs over its safety and if there might be any terrible outcomes on the pores and skin, leaving the character with troubles to deal with because of receiving the therapy. This is also real for red light remedy. There are many specific safety measures to recall whilst beginning treatments using purple slight treatment and one among a kind sorts of slight remedy. People who had pores and pores and skin most cancers or is treating this form of cancer need to keep away from moderate treatment as it is able to reason troubles in their very very own skin. Another circumstance is systemic lupus erythematosus, wherein the usage of red remedy isn't honestly useful. Those who do now not have those illnesses in their scientific records will no longer usually show off pores and skin-based totally definitely side results. It is crucial to offer adequate coverage of the skin in regions meant to get hold of the crimson moderate remedy. However, the regions that could not gather the remedy need to be prevented. During the remedy, appropriate material or covers want to be used to avoid permeation of mild into areas that need to not be receiving the crimson mild remedy. The appropriate garb want to additionally be used by the person administering the remedy because of the truth it may cause damage to the man or woman giving the remedy in a manner that isn't meant. If you have got end up the red moderate treatment in a spa putting or a health practitioner's workplace, lab coats and similar apparel are typically utilized by the man or woman offering the remedy to cowl uncovered pores and pores and pores and skin as it isn't always meant for them to acquire the pink mild. This moreover lets in block any incoming rays that could affect your vision with prolonged exposure.

Light remedy that most effective involves seen light wherein we're uncovered to on a regular foundation is normally taken into consideration secure. There are very uncommon times in which mild treatment ought to be decreased and stopped, and it varies relying at the individual and the extent of remedy they are receiving. Red mild remedy can be misconstrued as having the same kind of risky effects at the pores and skin as tanning beds. Red light remedy is considered to be secure and nicely-tolerated through most folks which can be taken into consideration to be in suitable fitness without a underlying situations that can be affected in a terrible manner thru crimson slight remedy. Unlike salon tanning beds which can be traditionally used to reveal the melanin in your skin in which it's far produced without a doubt, purple mild therapy remedies do no longer hire the use of ultraviolet (UV) rays which might be harmful, and might result to damaged pores and pores and skin. UV rays are also recognized to motive pores and pores and pores and skin cells to mutate. Red slight treatment, however, uses seen mild this is on the stop of the spectrum. It is just like infrared slight, and it makes use of infrared light sometimes as nicely. This type of mild is absorbed into the pores and pores and skin and is belief for its advantages to the frame further to your fitness. Tanning beds were known to accelerate the development of pores and pores and skin most cancers because of the UV rays which can be used within the remedy. When you're considering red slight remedy, recollect that it uses the safest form of mild on the spectrum in desire to the tanning beds we have got grown familiar with, and which use volatile rays that can harm your pores and skin and potentially cause pores and skin most cancers.

Short-Term Side Effects

Sometimes, purple mild remedy makes use of LED moderate, which is truely an observable mild that can be filtered to allow simplest a selected wavelength of slight via. When used for pink moderate treatment, LED mild frequently has no negative aspect consequences. Many research have established that, more regularly than no longer, folks that participate in receiving crimson mild therapy do no longer experience any element effects aside from the supposed consequences of the remedy. If, for some motive,undesirable issue consequences arise, those results are regularly trivial and do no longer remaining very prolonged. The only responses to purple slight remedy which have been recorded as potential side effects are:

• Headaches. Users can also revel in headaches, particularly even as the purple light remedy is being applied to the pinnacle or face.

• Eyestrain. This is likewise commonplace when there may be no protection worn at a few stage in the remedy, and the eyes are overexposed to the purple moderate. Eyestrain may additionally moreover arise if the therapy is being applied to areas of the pinnacle or face.

• Irritability. This is possible whilst we're overexposed to nice sorts of mild and is likewise not unusual if we are overexposed to daylight hours. It is probable simply a completely quick temper shift. Once you are uncovered on your normal levels of slight, your body has the possibility to readjust and you will enjoy much much less irritable.

These undesirable results are commonly created with the brightness from the mild used on this kind of remedy. You might also moreover find out the mild to be too excessive, especially on the identical time as trying out the red mild remedy for the first time. To lessen probabilities of experiencing terrible aspect results of red slight therapy, you need to keep away from staring into the source of mild immediately, specifically whilst laser is used. Another manner to avoid the ones horrific results is to position on prescribed eye safety. This applies extra importantly at the equal time as you administer the red mild remedy to your self at home. In addition, you need to are searching for medical recommendation in case you are considering making use of crimson mild therapy to your self when you have been diagnosed with a bipolar sickness. You have to observe that, in uncommon instances, it's far been recognized to purpose mania in sufferers which have this preexisting scenario in the past.

Since infrared moderate is likewise a shape of thermal power, now not like LED mild, the usage of it in red mild treatment can be much more likely to bring about those symptoms and symptoms. Side results of this kind of moderate can glaringly be related to overheating problems, that could motive the pores and pores and skin to burn. This can be a thermal burn, which isn't the same as the kind of burn that is skilled in a tanning mattress with UV bulbs. This type of burn will no longer cause most cancers; it's far in reality a minimal inflammation of the pores and skin that might be to move away as quickly as treated successfully and taken care of properly. In addition, if the pores and skin is overexposed, the remedy in that region have to be discontinued till it has time to heal. Overheating the pores and pores and skin cells may warp the cell's capability to repair DNA successfully, making it greater vulnerable to mutations initiated thru different influences. You need to be aware about burning the pores and pores and skin, and you could be secure via sticking to the remedy frequency endorsed for you. You want to furthermore preserve an agreeable spacebetween you and the tool that administers the infrared light. To do away with chance altogether, you have to severely bear in thoughts the usage of simplest LED as your purple moderate remedy slight deliver.

Eye Health with Red Light Therapy

As stated above, it's far essential that you appearance a ways from the mild deliver while going thru purple mild treatment. This is a stable way to undergo the way, despite the truth that the form of moderate is considered commonly stable for exposition. To extraordinary shield your eyes, you have to be sporting appropriate eye safety. There are many splendid forms of eye protection that you could use so that you can make certain which you are protected at the identical time as administering red mild treatment. If you are using a purple mild supply that is infrared, keep away from going close to the deliver of mild. An infrared moderate supply that has a >1500nm wavelength will no longer have an impact on the retina negatively, but it is able to purpose impairment to the lens and cornea that is probably eternal. Some people do not take their eye health severely sufficient, so it's miles critical to pay very near hobby for your eyes even as you're going via a form of treatment that may reason ability damage to them. If you are clever approximately your software application of red mild treatment and you are the use of the right eye safety, you do not need to worry about purple mild treatment negative your eyes.

Sometimes, it's far even viable to use red slight treatment to deal with tremendous types of eye conditions. These are remedies that need to be using purple moderate satisfactory, and no longer every special lighting at the spectrum. This is a form of remedy that want to be administered through a expert as it includes some issue very essential in your properly-being. It is crucial that is it finished proper each time, so you do now not harm your eyes or experience specific unfavourable outcomes, because of the truth it's miles very near your face and thoughts. Red slight remedy is taken into consideration stable for the eyes so long as it's miles achieved consistent with the suggestions which can be confident to help cope with the problem, but no longer purpose a few other terrible facet consequences. Be clever approximately your crimson slight treatment usage at the same time as it pertains in your eyes, and you want to don't have any hassle with using pink slight treatment for all your wishes. Like some thing else, in reality have in mind of what you're doing on your frame, and make certain which you are protecting yourself generally else.

There are typically no recorded lengthy-term issue outcomes on people who use purple mild therapy correctly. The simplest feasible element effect, in the end, is frequently attributed to the volatile use of the tool. This approach that, no longer the usage of the device nicely may also motive the pores and pores and skin tissues to overheat. While LED property on this remedy launch best a hint warm temperature, infrared light can also furthermore produce a tremendous deal of thermal energy. Some tissues in our frame can be extra sensitive to the boom in temperature in contrast to others. Take phrase that this is moreover the case to your eyes. As previously stated, overheating the lens or cornea of your eye can positioned you at risk of eye conditions which include cataracts. On the possibility hand, this is especially now not going to give up result in case you operate LED lights as an possibility, and if you stay real to the remedy time table that is super for you and your situation.

There are not many recorded times of purple slight remedy having terrible aspect effects, so long as the remedy is run successfully and is executed within the parameters which might be prescribed by using doctors. It is one of the maximum stable era inside the clinical region in recent times; many human beings are benefitting from it, mainly considering there aren't many factor outcomes that could motive specific issues for them in the long run. People who do their studies beforehand see what purple slight remedy can do for them, and that they may be able to use it for some of ailments they face. There are increasingly subjects that purple mild therapy can cope with, for this reason, it has grow to be increasingly more famous over the years. You are the handiest person who in truth knows how to attend to yourself, so it is critical so as to do as a incredible deal research as viable in advance than getting red slight treatment finished. You are within the proper location to begin your research with this e-book. We desire that this has helped lead you to a selection – we nice provide you with the high-quality information to make the nice selection for your health. We wish which you discover your self taking walks down the route of statistics the pink slight remedy and its advantages, which is probably as right for you as it changed into for others who skilled its advantages earlier than you.

Skin Issues with Red Light Therapy

Similar to the types of problem consequences that red moderate treatment may additionally show off, there aren't many recorded pores and pores and skin issues that have resulted from purple mild treatment. Skin issues are by and large said from the usage of infrared moderate therapy, because it motives the thermal warm temperature to heat up the skin, causing redness and contamination which can be normally now not durable and is with out trouble treatable. Despite this truth, it would now not be a horrible idea to put on sunscreen in a few unspecified time within the future of your red mild remedy treatments, especially if you are exposing alot of bare pores and pores and skin to the moderate. This would possibly assist to lessen the amount of publicity at the top layers of your skin, causing the crimson mild treatment to have an effect on handiest the regions in which you are trying to address. It is amazing to apprehend that you are capable of find a minimally-invasive remedy that has only a few side consequences and only can offer consequences that you desire. Also, it may assist with many amazing forms of body troubles that you will be experiencing. It is critical that you defend the pores and skin inside the regions that you aren't treating so that you can manipulate the quantity of exposure you get whilst the remedy is being administered. If you preserve the crimson slight remedy at once within the region wherein you are trying to deal with, you may no longer feel any horrible component outcomes in your pores and pores and skin. You will, but, be able to control in which the remedy goes, so that you have to be seeing outcomes earlier than expected than in case you reveal multiple areas of the frame to the remedy simultaneously. If the purple light remedy is being administered throughout multiple areas, it'll now not paintings as tough on on the meant place because it otherwise must.

Red light remedy is fairly specific from the alternative varieties of remedies, specially the ones which can be orally administered, i.E., medicine. Medication continuously comes with aspect effects that might likely final lengthy and can motive even more problems even as all you are trying to do is repair a trouble. There is often a lengthy listing of things that you need to be cautious for while taking many awesome drugs, and it regularly reasons more tension than it's miles nicely well worth. This is why humans are leaning extra toward crimson mild treatment than some other treatment, because of the close to to non-existent detail outcomes of the remedy. Treatments should now not include risky aspect results, and we are capable of get results that we need through red moderate remedy while not having to fear about harming ourselves even more while all we preference is to decorate our health and outer appearance. Red mild treatment is terrific for dad and mom that don't usually visit the clinical medical doctors for treatment as it reasons an excessive amount of anxiety. Red slight therapy may be administered at domestic, and, in stable situations, it could be surely as powerful due to the reality the administrative center treatments. Just preserve in thoughts all of the information you have got had been given positioned out from this e-book. In unique, you need to maintain your remedy inside the LED mild spectrum because of the reality this is the area this is the least probable to motive any pores and skin situations or awful factor effects that some can also moreover enjoy with the alternative slight spectrums.

Red Light Therapy and Cancer

Effective and guided use of purple moderate remedy is not acknowledged to cause any shape of most cancers if LED slight is administered. If you have got had any form of most cancers, mainly pores and skin maximum cancers, it is advocated which you avoid using purple slight remedy altogether. In addition, relying on the shape of most cancers, you want to as a minimum avoid the place wherein the most cancers is gift. Red mild remedy has the functionality to make cancers worse counting on the slight that is administered, however it isn't always recognized to motive most cancers in already wholesome people. There have been studies carried out to look if red slight remedy can virtually help cope with extraordinary types of cancers, but experts have yet to decide if it may cope with cancer, and they normally endorse keeping off it in case you do have most cancers. Studies have now not decided if purple slight treatment can assist maximum cancers, however it has proven that intense degrees of pink mild therapy the usage of slight that isn't especially LED ought to make cancers worse, specifically in case you aren't listening to what is being administered and are overexposing your self to the slight. It is critical to recognize what tissues beneath the primary layers of pores and pores and skin can be exposed to the purple mild on the identical time as it is being administered, to appearance if there are cells that could in all likelihood become cancerous, or the triumphing most cancers cells can absorb the moderate and mutate the cells to make maximum cancers unfold.

Ultimately, it isn't assured that red slight remedy can purpose most cancers, neither is it assured that crimson mild treatment will make cancers worse. Although this is the choice up to now, it does no matter the fact that make experience to keep away from crimson slight remedy on regions of the body wherein cancer have become or remains present to keep away from any viable complications a number of the pink slight treatment and maximum cancers. Cancer is a scary factor, and it has end up increasingly more of a danger with particular styles of medical treatments. Thankfully, red slight remedy remains considered one of the most secure technology accessible these days, because it isn't always identified to cause maximum cancers. Knowing how to attend to your self even as you are looking to attain crimson light remedy is your great wager. You want to accordingly keep away from the times of publicity that you do not want to experience. It is safe to mention that administering purple moderate treatment onto yourself will now not cause most cancers, and this is the critical problem to recognize whilst you're thinking about some thing new for the number one time. It is as lots as you to do as a good deal research as possible in advance than starting any sort of remedy. Moreover, it is practical to attempting to find recommendation from a systematic professional in advance than the use of pink moderate remedy because of the truth scientific doctors are the superb source of data to answer any questions you can have.

You can entire this financial disaster information that red light treatment is a safe approach for your dreams, and which you do no longer need to fear approximately having to cope with any lousy facet consequences on the aspect of it. Be advantageous to observe any rules and suggestions which might be set by using way of the scientific physician you're consulting regarding your treatment. Follow all guidelines to make sure you're exposed fine to the prescribed amount of red slight for the durations of time which have been encouraged. Do not set your very personal quantity of moderate for use because of the truth this is while you could likely motive more damage than right on your self. Be clever and steady, and you have to now not have any issues in some unspecified time inside the destiny of your use of purple slight treatment. Red slight therapy has acquired no longer whatever however right critiques up to now, and it indicates that crimson slight is a few thing that might help everybody with our medical troubles. It might be interesting to look, within the years yet to come, what crimson mild treatment can treatment. Think about this and be aware about what you're reading on-line due to the fact purple slight remedy can be mentioned in a terrible mild through people who might not have had the top notch testimonies with it. Make sure that those money owed are coming from reviewed documentation and also your clinical professionals to ensure you've got got turn out to be the nice records possible. You can see so many remarkable benefits from pink light treatment, and we are hoping that this financial ruin has calmed any of your crucial issues that you may have had approximately pink mild remedy.

## Chapter 4: Recommended Dosage And Guidance

The reason of this financial disaster is to remind you which ones you need to heed all warnings not to overdo your remedies. While crimson moderate remedy is normally taken into consideration very stable, questioning that "extra is higher" and then overdoing your exposure instances or huge sort of treatments will in reality lower the effectiveness of the remedy. This should remind you that it is essential to recognize and cling to the overall suggestions which can be obtainable for pink slight treatment dosing. It must additionally be stated that crimson mild treatment dosage can be complicated due to the fact it is a complex technology that has a massive style of gadgets and unique doses. And those have been applied in precise studies, not unusual body area handled, and the forms of remedy administered. You have to moreover maintain in thoughts the desires of the treatment, in addition to the great frame troubles you are trying to cope with. Because of these complex issues, one-of-a-type people from time to time have precise views on the appropriate dosage. Some human beings most effective advise very low doses administered with lasers. Others propose inside the course of using lasers altogether. Others who propose large doses expect that it isn't possible to overdose on crimson mild therapy. So, there are a number of people who do not take delivery of as true with every awesome at the finer information of dosage. With all of those in thoughts, bear in mind that there can be a desired consensus on what degrees of doses are powerful for all, and it comes from the vicinity's maximum valid professionals in purple mild treatment. The famous dosing recommendations we're capable of provide are imagined to be used with LED panel fashion mild gadgets.

So, permit us to do a recap on what we have were given referred to to this point: If you want to have an powerful red light treatment session, you want to first use an effective dose. An effective dose requires a mild that is fairly powerful, because of this it has a great level of energy density. Next, you could need a slight which can deal with a large vicinity of the body abruptly. Then, you can want an facts of the maximum relevant period of time the usage of the mild to get the right total dose. Too small a dose will now not provide you with the results which you are searching out. If your dose is simply too sturdy, you may get minimal to no effects as well. You need to locate the proper dose for all your goals so you get the top-rated dose on every occasion you administer the red moderate therapy. The strength density of mild should have an impact on the pinnacle-excellent degree of mild wanted for powerful remedy.

Distance from the Light

Power density is the quantity of power that is emitted in a place. In greater smooth phrases, in case you are using a light to your body with an area this is approximately 50cm with the aid of 40cm, and the light which you are the usage of is 200W, then you have spherical 100mW/cm2 due to the fact the energy density. This is a notable power density for use in the remedy. Beyond clean calculations, there are a few things that may make a easy calculation more complex. You will first need to reflect onconsideration on your distance a ways from the mild. You need to look at that the energy density of mild decreases considerably as you skip further far from the mild supply. This manner that you could get the best dose of the mild by way of way of being within just a few inches of it. If you're greater than 3 toes far from the mild, you can get little to no impact as it will not get anywhere near below the ground of the skin in which you are purported to be treating. However, this does not commonly suggest that being within the route of the mild is incredible. You ought to make it a desired rule that being inches faraway from the moderate supply is terrific, simply to shield your self toward any exposure to EMFs. This additionally applies to all of the virtual gadgets in your existence. You must hold a stage of 6 to 36 inches' distance from the device always. It is essential to understand that the space from the mild dramatically influences the dose wherein your cells get hold of the purple moderate treatment.

Light Wavelengths
Depending at the tool, first-class gadgets emit all of the mild output/wattage in what are called "effective recovery wavelengths", and others also can emit simplest a part of their general wattage in restoration wavelengths. This approach that the complete wattage is super 20-60%, and is not the greatest healing wavelength. This is a few element that contributes to the factors of the dose. This

may want to make calculations pretty complicated, relying on the moderate supply that is getting used. We recognize that specific wavelengths come from numerous kinds of slight, so it is for your gain to searching for out doctors and devices that emit LED moderate if you need to acquire treatment inside the exceptional restoration wavelength. It is important to parent out what is the best mild wavelengths, due to the fact you do no longer want to over or underexpose your pores and pores and skin to the crimson mild. Remember that underexposure may not deem the treatment powerful, on the identical time as overexposure would probably create unwanted side outcomes, and in the end, you cannot see the consequences you are looking forward to from your crimson slight therapy. Once you determine out your preferred wavelength for what you are trying to cope with, it's going to assist you discover the proper dosage and the proper device that you want as a manner to get the maximum from your destiny crimson mild treatment treatments.

Claimed Wattage vs. Actual Wattage

There is a distinction a number of the claimed wattage and the actual wattage electricity output of a moderate. Claimed wattage is what the moderate is rated for, and the real is the real intensity of the moderate emitted. It is usually understood that a mild bulb emits a energy density this is about 25-50% decrease than the claimed wattage would possibly normally suggest. So, despite the fact that we've the calculation above, with this records, it makes it greater of a concept or a suggestion. You do not understand the real light depth output of the light you get till you genuinely take some time to diploma it. If you are interested by gaining knowledge of more approximately locating out the way to degree the real output of a light, there are numerous first rate assets on line that will help you decide this, relying on the shape of moderate you are going for walks with. It can also assist to hold in mind that actual moderate output is form of 50% lower than what the organizations are claiming.

Size of the Device and the Size of the Treatment Area

One of the maximum essential topics to be aware about is the dimensions of the device and the size of the location you are trying to address. Even if you have a tool that is effective sufficient to create a useful effect, it may be too small for the region you're searching for to deal with. So, in spite of the fact that the tool has the proper electricity density, it may only be a few inches in circumference, so it simplest emits mild over a totally small a part of your frame. If you are trying to deal with big regions of the frame, this makes the light which you have extraordinarily inefficient and often very time-consuming. You want to discover a device this is big sufficient to cowl the location you are attempting to deal with and has the capability to supply the proper quantity of mild wished a terrific manner to make a distinction. Overall, the device desires to emit the proper type of slight above a nice strength density, and it desires to be at the proper wavelengths. It moreover ought to be physical big enough to emit the proper amount of light on the appropriate a part of your body. Moreover, it must be used from a right distance some distance from the location of your frame that you are treating.

So now we need to apprehend, for how long we must show ourselves to the slight to get the nice remedy? For skin troubles and one in every of a kind extra superficial problems which may be in the direction of the floor of the pores and pores and skin, there are a few things we should realize: For the ones styles of conditions, we want a low commonplace dose to every location of the pores and skin. There is some indication that decrease electricity densities may be greater greatest for treating the pores and skin than higher energy densities. Do no longer permit this make you trust you studied that decrease strength lights are desirable; better energy lighting although have a miles higher gain due to the fact they permit you to be in addition a long way from the slight and concurrently deal with a bigger location of your frame with an most suited dosage of moderate. Smaller lighting are stated to be more inefficient and time-consuming, and they may be very limited within the sorts of treatments they may be used for.

In assessment to this, in case you are attempting to deal with deep tissue issues, you may want a larger dose and a higher electricity density for the most maximum beneficial effects in your frame. In preferred, you could need to have the mild thousands inside the direction of your frame with a much better depth. This is what you'll want to deliver an maximum outstanding dose of mild into the deeper factors of your pores and skin tissues.

With pores and pores and skin and floor treatments, you may need to be in addition some distance from the mild. This helps decrease the mild depth and cover a bigger region of the body. In addition, this can give you an commonplace lower dosage to your body. With deep tissue troubles, you need to be within the course of the slight. This then will increase the slight depth and the general dose obtained.

To make this extra specific and sensible, the following are a few pointers that you can comply with:

For Skin Issues
Assuming that you are using the recommended lighting fixtures on your pores and pores and skin troubles and body troubles, the fundamental usage hints for you is someplace among 1 - 4 minutes for round 12 inches a long way from the location. For skin issues, it is advocated going at least 12 inches far

from the tool; with troubles on deep tissue, you need to be closer and characteristic a higher strength density. You moreover have the choice of 1.Five - 5 minutes and an 18-inch distance from the device. In addition, you can administer the treatment in 2 - 8 minutes at a distance of 24 inches from your body, counting on the sort of problem that you are handling. If you have got come to be a slight this is endorsed, this is certainly all you want to understand concerning the period of time which you should be uncovered to the mild.

For Deep Tissue

For issues in deep tissue, which consist of in the muscle, ligament, bone, tendons, the mind, and organs, you may want a much better dose than formerly described. This technique that you'll want a effective device, and the distance amongst you and the tool must be round 6 to 12 inches, it's contrary to treating pores and pores and skin problems. This is how you'll get the maximum high-quality dose of mild for deep tissue troubles. Depending on how grave the trouble is, you may want to deliver the moderate toward your body. The better the general dose you operate, the better the tool will deliver results. You can gain maximum green outcomes and adequate recuperation doses on deep tissue problems. For use at the thoughts, this will require a higher dose as well, as it takes a pretty immoderate dose for sufficient moderate to penetrate through the cranium and be efficaciously introduced to the mind. General tips for deep tissues beneath the skin embody the instances illustrated beneath: Using mild 6 inches some distance from the pores and pores and skin amongst 2 - 7 minutes in line with vicinity is the right dose range. You can also do it for five - 10 mins from 12 inches away. Generally, you want to not get farther than 12 inches even as you're managing deep tissue.

If you pick out out a high-quality tool than what is recommended, you can should do your very private calculations the use of the equations which can be provided. You can really paintings on the ones calculations your self, information that it is best pretty simple math. Just maintain in thoughts that the actual wattage is usually a bargain decrease than what the producer claims, and that is authentic for the diverse lighting fixtures available. So, in case your calculations are based totally on the claimed wattage in desire to the actual measurements, your calculations will probable be off through a massive margin because of this. Just keep in mind that greater is not continually higher.

There is some issue known as "biphasic dose reaction", because of this that doing an excessive amount of of the treatment can truly result in lesser benefit than what you can count on. In pink slight treatment, you have to no longer count on that little is good and additional is better. All this would lead you to do is decrease the benefits of your crimson slight therapy, and you can must do extra of the remedy in some time so you can get the proper consequences. You need to furthermore keep in thoughts that during case your health is currently compromised, this kingdom may additionally need to make you greater fragile. In addition, you may not be capable of tolerate alot of slight. If you're a healthful, more younger individual who overdoses on mild remedy, you could not be conscious some factor. An sick character, but, must study the horrible results and often revel in fatigued as a prevent result. Ill people are typically a bargain an awful lot a good deal much less tolerant, and their our bodies have a lower threshold for overdoing treatment as compared to a person who is notably greater healthful and greater younger. So, as a reminder to actually every person who is in very horrible health, it is actually critical first of all very low doses to ensure your body can tolerate it first. Then, you may slowly boom your dose in the following days or maybe weeks or as you be aware fit. So you can artwork your way in the direction of the range this is useful for you.

Overdosing on Red Light Therapy
As formerly noted, there may be a issue in pink mild remedy called the "biphasic dose reaction". This method that too little red slight therapy will no longer provide a whole lot advantage, and too much may negate a gain. It is critical to get the dosage right and within the advocated range. You are not assisting your self in any way via dosing higher than the advocated guidelines. The thoughts of the biphasic dose reaction is defined within the Arndt-Schulz law, it's a regulation that dates decrease once more to the surrender of the 19th century. Back then, Schulz analyzed the hobby of numerous varieties of poisoning, and he showed that in very lower doses, all of these are without a doubt lightly stimulatory. When the height is reached, however, an increase inside the dosage must in

addition suppresses the effect till a volatile effect is eventually reached. It is likewise important to notice that it's miles plenty less complicated to overdose floor tissues in assessment to the deeper tissues. The maximum green dose for the skin may be reached in mere seconds, and it is very smooth for humans to apply the devices 2 to 3 times longer than it is right. People are wondering that doing greater outcomes in higher consequences, but they will be sincerely starting to negate the benefits within the machine of doing this.

There is an example of this outside of purple mild remedy, and it is taken from bodily exercise: In small and slight doses, exercise is truely connected with many health benefits. But, as we recognize, with folks who over exercising, it may absolutely reason a tremendous deal of damage. It is not uncommon to check about marathon runners losing useless from coronary coronary heart assaults or female athletes losing their fertility after over-workout. Anyone who has overdone it in terms of workout is aware about that fatigue is a completely common problem impact. Overtraining in athletes effects in fatigue, despair, complications, insomnia, and weakened immune structures. Exercise is incredibility powerful, but only while it is finished in the proper portions for our body. Too a good deal exercise will probably have terrible outcomes. If you overdo it to the intense, you could damage your cells.

Fortunately, red mild treatment is more steady and has heaps a whole lot much less potential to cause harm while you overdo it than both sunlight hours or over-exercise. Therefore, this makes pink mild treatment extraordinarily safe. People can use purple slight remedy for many years and take transport of as actual with that it's far very tough to overdo it in a manner that negates the blessings. If you overdo it barely, you will now not probably see the terrible outcomes. Many people will not even phrase facet consequences even though overdosing occurs regularly. If you hugely overdo a dose, however, it is commonplace to experience fatigued and increase a slight headache. That is generally as terrible as maximum human beings get. Someone who's greater fragile, and who's present method purple mild treatment will have a look at greater big fatigue at the same time as they'll be overdosing with red mild remedy. Basically, however, there can be very restricted functionality for facet results with overdosing on red moderate remedy in evaluation to over-exercise and overdoing it with sun publicity.

Therefore, it's miles crucial to pay attention to how you sense after each dose of pink slight remedy. If you take a look at that you are beginning to experience fatigued after your doses, that is often a signal that you are overdoing the dose a piece compared to what has been encouraged. You want to recollect reducing the dose, and your hassle will probable be solved. You can consider it this manner: If you get in reality sore and tired after doing a clearly excessive exercising, may you determined that the exercising is terrible for you, as it makes you feel horrible, and which you have to surrender? Or, are you more likely to take into account the reality that there are research available displaying that exercising is beneficial for your health? If you are in truth worn-out and infected, you need to dial down the intensity to offer your body a harm in advance than persevering with workout at that degree. You can usually do sporting activities which are more suitable on your frame kind and fitness diploma.

Ultimately, it's miles great to seek advice from a systematic expert on what dose, exposure time, and degree are super for you and the issue you are attempting to cope with. Even if you are attempting to do those strategies at home, it's far essential which you paintings with a manual so that you aren't unnecessarily overexposing your self to purple slight. If you need to make sure that the advocated doses are proper for you, you could generally speak to the calculations furnished to ensure which you are operating the red mild remedy at the best diploma. If you are involved about overexposing your self inside the path of your red moderate remedy, you need to start at the bottom stop of the spectrum so that you can slowly constructing up your body to the remedy, and you may enjoy extra snug within the degree of pink moderate which you are receiving. You recognize your non-public frame and what's satisfactory for you, so if you revel in that the encouraged dose is too much or too little for you, paintings with a expert to appearance if reducing or developing the dose is first-rate for you and your fitness. The closing thing you may need to do is create a horrible effect in region of a amazing one.

# Chapter 5: Professional Vs. Home Equipment And Choosing The Right Equipment

Choosing amongst getting your pink slight remedy finished with the useful resource of a professional in an office setting and getting professional grade machine to apply at home genuinely is based upon on your alternatives and if you have any issues with going to the clinical medical doctors. Red moderate treatment is now supplied in spa-like settings, so this allows humans who've anxiety over going to the physician's place of job. Receiving purple slight remedy in a spa, as a substitute an place of business is a exquisite way for humans to lighten up and be cushty even as they're receiving their treatment because it usually is a completely calming environment. This is probably the proper manner to move, especially at the beginning of your remedies. With this, you have the opportunity to analyze from a professional who is expert in giving the pink mild therapy. In addition, you can pick out to do the therapy at home as quickly as you have the right tool that allows you to acquire the equal amount of dosage as you'll get preserve of on the spa. Depending for your budget, it's miles important to decide out which road is extraordinary for you, so that you are not going to pay for a tool this is too difficult to use or which you aren't high-quality how to use and end up overexposing yourself to the purple slight. In this monetary wreck, we are able to provide you with the positives and negatives of every research and help you choose the right machine based mostly on the type of treatment you are searching for to gather.

Professional and Equipment for Home Use
Not only is purple light remedy being provided in spa-like settings, however moreover tanning shops throughout the kingdom. The red slight therapy is

administered via the same shape of lay-down tanning mattress you often see in the ones tanning stores. However, it is handiest the use of the LED pink mild in region of the UV slight bulbs in conventional tanning beds. These make it accessible to get your crimson mild remedy in this shape of placing due to the truth tanning stores are frequently positioned on each corner and it does not need waiting time like in a conventional medical doctor's place of work putting. Plus, you have the introduced benefit of being in a private room so you can experience snug getting the treatment.

Dermatologists, aestheticians, and different licensed pores and pores and skin care professionals use severa LED machine in their remedy rooms simply so they will be capable of accommodate and deal with remarkable areas of the body. Most artwork with the face and higher body, for the purpose that people will go to those specialists for anti-developing antique pain and pimples treatment. Given the type of remedy they will be administering, there are one-of-a-kind varieties of device they're able to use relying on the dimensions of the affected region. It is crucial that they use the right-sized system due to the reality if it is too small, it will no longer be as powerful, and if it's far too huge, you may be overexposed to the pink moderate in areas that do not want the treatment. Most medical experts are skilled in administering crimson slight treatment, and they may be completely privy to which device is first-rate on your goals. In addition, they recognize a way to administer it effectively and correctly for you to see the excellent consequences. This is why we additionally advise that maximum humans start in a expert putting because of the reality then you may be in a position to talk thru the whole method with a certified professional. They can be capable of deal with any problems you can have and provide you with the right treatment plan based totally on your goals.

LightStim creates two one among a type styles of devices for experts that modify in duration and form. They are each geared inside the course of treating anti-developing antique pimples and pain. The first one is a expert 2-panel mild that lets in for hands-unfastened software program program and a completely programmable timer just so the professional can carry out unique offerings concurrently at the same time as administering the mild treatment. It consists of hinged panels so it is able to deal with the edges of the body and face that are not continuously on hand via the usage of manner of diverse varieties of gadgets for crimson mild treatment. It moreover has an articulating arm in order that it may conform properly to the consumer's remedy area without any more paintings or stress. LightStim additionally created a hand-held slight that looks just like the thing and shape of a handheld showerhead. It has the identical expert electricity as the two-panel moderate, however it's far portable and comes in a cheap duration, so it is easy to apply. It moreover has a conformable control, in case you are searching out remedy in a small constricted vicinity of the frame and want to hold the red mild an extended way from close by regions. LightStim is likewise accredited for domestic use so you may additionally additionally have an lots less high-priced professional-grade era in the comfort of your home.

There are also expert facial masks which might be to be had in place of business treatments and domestic use. Deesse Professional is a maker of one of the crimson mild face masks which have been made well-known through film celeb aestheticians everywhere in the global. Deesse noticed the recognition of the face mask surge as quickly as celebrities began speakme approximately how remarkable the technology labored. They created a greater lots much less luxurious choice for individuals who favored to try out the mask at home. Chrissy Teigen modified into one film famous man or woman that first commenced out sharing that she emerge as the usage of one of the crimson light remedy masks at home, and soon it took off, and the market boomed. The proper expert mask that come to be created supplied different moderate settings and protected a couple of shade moderate remedy alternatives. It become promoting for over $1500! With this newly-created single slight masks costing most effective round $350, it's far an low-cost alternative for every experts and those trying to acquire the treatment at home. The mild masks is especially to be used in the course of the face, and may help with anti-developing older and zits pores and pores and pores and skin issues too. This is what the mask are maximum broadly used for, and having it in a centered shape that works near the face is splendid because of the fact that is the sort of remedy you're looking for at the same time as going for walks with wrinkles and pimples. These mask often emit a low dose of crimson slight remedy, and at the same time as used as directed, you will no longer have any foreseeable horrible aspect effects as however the fact that it is so near your pores and pores and skin, it will now not damage you.

From Dr. Dennis Gross Skincare, they have got created a tool this is precise for the vicinity throughout the eyes. They have produced the SpecraLiteEyeCare Pro, and it ranges from round $159. This is an anti-developing antique device that enables boom collagen manufacturing and enables lessen the advent of amazing traces and wrinkles throughout the eyes. It is good for hyperpigmentation, growing older pores and skin, crow's feet, and lack of pores and pores and skin firmness, first-class lines, and wrinkles. This tool will help you advantage extra extra youthful looking eyes, as this is one region of our face that maximum normally show growing older, specially in ladies. Many girls begin receiving expert treatments for the location around their eyes as fast as they see wrinkles. Because crow's toes are commonplace as we age, and it's also related to developing older in society, ladies will be inclined to get remedies finished that help correct it. This product contains seventy LED lighting fixtures that have a entire range of recovery lighting fixtures, and it additionally has a fingers-loose layout, so you are able to get professional outcomes within the office in addition to in the comfort of your own home. This product is capable of penetrate into the deep layers of your pores and pores and skin that allows you to decorate your collagen levels and easy out the advent of first-class strains and wrinkles. The key advantages of this product are that it firms the pores and pores and pores and skin and increases its density, all whilst moreover middle of the night out the pores and pores and skin's texture. It is right for pores and pores and skin kinds which might be pimples-inclined, oily, dry, aggregate, ordinary, touchy, and mature skin types. It is constant to be used for all pores and skin types and a long term, as long as you are taking the critical precautions to defend your eyes whilst doing the treatment.

PlatinumLED Therapy Lights has advanced a line of crimson mild remedy lighting fixtures that variety in duration and LED electricity elegance to provide a extensive style of gadgets that might goal special regions of the body depending on the scale and location. The four merchandise they produce are: The BIO-3 hundred, BIO-450, BIO-six hundred, and BIO-900. As you may possibly guess, the range related to the name of the product is likewise in which it falls within the LED power beauty. The BIO-three hundred and -450 are remarkable for focused regions, at the equal time because the -six hundred and -

900 are for whole frame remedies. Depending on the dimensions, it tiers from 2 to 5 cooling fanatics which can be built into the device so you can preserve to hold your body cool while the usage of the slight remedy. They all include recuperation-grade LED bulbs and function a ninety-degree lens beam attitude. Each buy comes with a mounting hardware, door setting kit, sunglasses and a remedy-accomplice app that may be used in your cellphone to permit you to understand what treatment grade to apply and the way prolonged you want to be exposed to the light. It comes with a 3-yr assure insurance, and all the devices are FDA-permitted. At 12" mild meter, the -3 hundred has a 40 three" x 33" footprint, the -450 has a forty three" x 35", the -600 has a 60" x 33" footprint, and the -900 has a 60" x 37" footprint. Depending at the frame therapy you're desiring to be finished, that is a incredible preference to have both in the administrative center and at domestic. With this, you can cowl wider

areas for treatment, and you can moreover keep it at the again of a door, so you do now not must worry approximately it staying upright or protective it to your arms as you're receiving remedy. This tool is likewise brilliant for your joints because you could variety your distance nearer or farther far from the moderate and although revel in all the advantages of red mild treatment, and you most effective want to get one tool to achieve this at home.

Sharper Image has released a LED Hand Pain Relief Mitten that makes use of a clean mitt and red slight LEDs embedded in it to control red slight therapy to centered regions of the arms and wrist. It modified into designed to cope with hand pain and stiffness with clinical-grade infrared LED lighting. It enables with arthritis pain and distinct ailments which might be related to the hands. It can also assist with Carpal Tunnel Syndrome, nerve accidents, repeating stress injuries, in addition to special aches and pains. It is easy to use because it lays flat on any floor and does now not require you to keep it at any element in the therapy session. It is a large length, so it's far flexible to match each male and lady hand sizes. It is a treatment that is non-invasive, non-ablative and produces drug-loose pain comfort. It has been cleared with the beneficial aid of the FDA and is an OTC Class 2 scientific tool. It comes with an on/off switch and actually desires to be plugged into an AC outlet or a USB port for use. Treatment time takes approximately 20 minutes, so it isn't always a few issue as a manner to absorb loads of area or time for your every day recurring, and you could get maintain of the treatment at the same time as additionally doing one of a kind responsibilities. It consists of each crimson and infrared LEDs, however you're incredible capable of see the purple moderate it produces because of the truth infrared slight can not be visible with the aid of using the human eye. The instructions on a way to apply are easy to comply with, and it's far furnished at an reasonably-priced fee factor of $a hundred 90.

Sharper Image has moreover launched the number one at-domestic professional LED lip treatment device. It uses powerful LED lighting to lessen and prevent wrinkles and creases within the perioral area. It skills 56 powerful LEDs that stimulate the manufacturing of collagen for plumper, greater more youthful looking lips. The tool furthermore enables with pores and skin tone and colour enhancement throughout the lip vicinity. The LED mild covers the whole lip location, and most effective calls for a 3-minute duration for treatment, and it can be used as a lot as five times every week for an 8- week duration. It has been medically established and clinically examined to be regular and herbal and now not the use of a thing consequences after treatment. This device is extra steady to use than receiving Botox remedies, which is likewise usually used for plumping the pores and skin during the lips to cause them to appear fuller and extra younger. Botox has an extended list of bad issue results, and pretty some human beings are finding out the difficult way that they're really allergic to the remedy and function had critical and occasionally deadly reactions to this type of remedy. Using crimson mild therapy is non-invasive and consists of no risk of allergic reactions, so it is safe to perform at domestic for added younger-looking lips in as low as 8 weeks. In addition, the outcomes are prolonged-lasting with the treatment. With Botox, it in the end wears off, and also you want to preserve to build up the treatment for a whole existence a excellent way to keep the popular outcomes.This can be disturbing for loads of human beings due to the fact, relying on wherein you drift for the remedy and who is acting it, you may get distinctive results every time. Also, regularly, you can get someone who isn't nicely-educated in administering it that may cause your lips to appearance uneven or have factor effects. You will now not want to worry approximately a whole lot of those in case you made a decision on red slight therapy as an opportunity.

DPL Flex has advanced a systematic-grade infrared mild pad that can be used at various locations on the body for pain comfort. It allows you recover from harm and eases the normal pains that we also can experience virtually from developing older and no longer being able to pass as an entire lot as we used to. This moderate securely boosts healing, stimulates the movement of blood in the body, relaxes your muscle tissue, and gets rid of all ache related to many bodily situations that every body face eventually in our lives. The remedy may be administered for up to 20 minutes, and you could feel immediately relief after the treatment. It has been categorized via FDA as an over-the-counter beauty 2 medical tool. It has a handy "wrap" function that suits the contours of various frame regions simply, with out a slipping or readjustment favored. It covers a remedy location of eight" x 5" inches, that is a fairly large location. It can penetrate deep into the tissue as well. This makes the device top notch for illnesses like arthritis, swelling within the ankle, pain of the decrease decrease returned, neuropathy, and tissue restore. It is also proper for assuaging sports activities sports activities accidents, sprains, and shoulder stiffness. It is a secure opportunity to ache drugs, minus the awful aspect consequences and the drug content cloth, as it's miles non-invasive. It is artificial to keep walking for years earlier than carrying out, and it comes with a one-twelve months guarantee, particularly on the USB port and cable. This product is to be had in at a barely higher charge point of $ hundred, however due to the fact you can use it on multiple regions of your body, it's far bendy and properly properly well really worth the investment. Typically, whilst we are injured, there are more than one components of our body wherein we enjoy ache. With this tool, you could address a couple of regions at a time at the same time as now not having to make journeys to the medical physician for a couple of remedies. Because it's far flexible, it's also very clean to keep. You do now not ought to fear about having bulky medical device around the residence due to the fact it's miles very smooth to keep in storage. This can in shape without issues in a linen cupboard, or it may be stored wherein you maintain your unique medical resources, as it's far the size of a small discipline. It is also tremendous to maintain in an area in that you have clean get right of get admission to to to to.

Similar to an entire lot of the expert scientific gadgets in locations much like the spa and doctors' places of work, this device additionally offers you the selection to purchase it for use at home. If you visit the spa and spot a tool which you pick out over the others, it would be easy for you to do research on that device and spot if it's far internal your finances to buy for use at domestic. At-domestic purple moderate remedy is becoming increasingly more famous – many medical device organizations are developing with extra moderen device all of the time. Because of this, it is a remarkable idea to keep your eye to be had available on the market to search for devices that help with the region of your challenge which you want to be handled. You can not flow wrong with both expert or at-domestic device – simply make sure you do the art work and appearance up everything in advance than buying them, so that you can ensure which you have turn out to be sincere device from official groups. This allows you to keep away from searching for defective machine which have the functionality to damage you in any manner. We however suggest which you start with professional treatments in advance than bringing your remedies home, so that you have the possibility to artwork with the tool in advance than you spend the coins for domestic use. Both options are much less expensive, and relying on what remedy you need, you are in all likelihood to discover a few issue that works properly and could offer you with the effects that you are searching out. We desire that this section of the e-book has given you an idea on what kind of tool to look for, and which you are probable to find some thing so one can offer you with the consequences you want at any factor in your lifestyles, each for beauty purposes or recuperation any pores and pores and pores and skin or ache troubles you are coping with. If you've got were given any questions associated with specific gadgets, we propose which you attain out to the groups that manufacture them, due to the fact they may be the excellent supply of records of their products. They need to be more than inclined that will help you in any way viable to ensure to procure the best care and have a fulfilling and professional enjoy operating with their corporation.

# Chapter 6: Why Eat Give Up End Result?

If you're a everyday eater of culmination with five to 7 kinds on your table each day, then you definitely're doing a awesome approach! A diet plan that doesn't embody quit stop end result isn't always a healthy weight loss program. Properly nourished humans are people who often consume stop result further to vegetables. In the equal manner, end result assist lower the threat of having ill. Why? Because end result are low in salt, low in fats, low in electricity, low in ldl cholesterol, and commonly unique assets of potassium, antioxidants (Vitamins C, A, and E), fiber, B-complicated, and folate. Their vitamins are quality at the identical time as every range is eaten sparkling and uncooked. But this doesn't suggest that cooked culmination aren't nutritious. It is only that the impact of the nourishing substances while heated isn't at its extraordinary.

The disappointing truth is that these days, purchasers are consuming smaller quantities of culmination. As a result, the dietary suggestions for healthful nutrients on the ones plant components aren't nicely met. According to the World Health Organization (WHO), 2.7 million lives might be saved each year if exceptional human beings eat more give up end result and greens. Likewise, the United States National Cancer Institute along side the World Health Organization associated the growing hazard and fee of cancers with the shortage of fruit and vegetable consumption.[1]Based on this opinion, the wonderful illness-curing outcomes of give up result which can be supported through manner of way of fitness restoration evidences need to be skilled. How? It is by way of using actually beginning to devour five to 9 servings of fruit types each day. The World Health Organization recommends no much less than 400g of end result every day (excluding potatoes and one of a kind starch-filled vegetation).[2]However, this recommended consumption is simply the minimal. Consumption varies counting on your location or u.S. Of the usa. On the opportunity hand, pick out the give up end result which might be full of the splendid health reaping benefits vitamins as cease end result range in vitamins.

"But why do many humans pay no immoderate interest to right consumption of cease end result even if they understand the gain the ones plant additives supply to the body?"

There are many factors that have an effect on terrible intake of end cease end result like availability, dependancy, fee, and the "I just don't find it impossible to resist" thoughts-set. If a person is not within the addiction of consuming fruits frequently, he is going to in no way take the advantages of consuming them seriously. There may be many excuses no longer like

115

if someone is oriented to each day intake of fruits from early years to maturity degree. But, a superb dependancy can be normal. Start it with a 21-day recurring of little by little eating fruit sorts and also you'll benefit with the change. Availability is also some other hindering element. Because of preoccupation, people have a propensity to buy precooked and processed food in area of purposely locating give up result in groceries and open markets. Others select to consume out and keep away from making prepared their very personal meals because of exhaustion. How do you oppose this? Try to save canned and easy fruits in the kitchen in which you could without troubles see them and consume proper away. Just accumulate enough quantity for intake, even though. Just the same, many people lose the interest of eating end result because of taste possibilities. Most humans assume that give up result are bland and dull to consume. With the peelings and all, the more strive would be too much and certainly as inconvenient as getting ready meals. The price of path is one of the maximum influential elements that prevent people from buying end result especially in horrible international places and their localities. If the costs of give up cease result are a whole lot less pricey, many may want to shop for them. Sadly, folks that extended to devour fruits regularly are the common people who may additionally as an alternative fill their stomachs with any food to be had and less expensive than bask in pricey end result. Other elements are the tempting tastes of junk food that human beings determine upon in desire to the healthy nutrient-packed natural food.

Fresh end result exceed in nutrients than food regimen dietary supplements bought in fitness shops. "Five quit end result each day preserve the contamination away!" If entire stop result do now not have any attraction to you, strive the pre-lessen and organized ones. Just 2 cups of end end result equivalent to 9 servings a day will make a big distinction!

Top Super Fruits

GUAVA
(Psidium Guajava)

Guava is a completely well-known tropical fruit because of its richness in Vitamin C. The fruit's shade stages from green to yellow green. The internal seedy crisp flesh is white or pink even as ripe. Guava's taste is specific, a bit like tartly sweet. It can develop big counting on its range and cultivation techniques. The fruit is available in a few unspecified time within the future of the 365 days except in some unspecified time in the future of summers. It is commonly grown as a outdoor fruit and is valued for its immoderate nutrients. The fruit with out issue suits to the magnificence of "splendid stop cease end result."

Nutrients in Guava

Guavas are an extraordinary deliver of carbohydrates and an notable deliver of Vitamin C and fiber. A guava offers to 3 times the quantity of Vitamin C than orange juice.

This is the nutrients precis of a cup of guava.

Note:If a particular nutrient isn't present, it does not usually imply that the fruit has none of it. It method that the nutrient's amount of hobby does not meet the rating tool standards.

Benefits of Guava

Guava is a totally super supply of antioxidant in Vitamin C this is 3 times extra than the day by day recommended consumption. The outer rind has greater Vitamin C content material fabric cloth than the flesh. Guava culmination are accurate opponents of maximum cancers. Eating the fruit regularly stops the formation of most cancers cells due to its excessive rate of Vitamin C and special antioxidants. It in particular protects the colon membranes, as a result stopping colon maximum cancers from happening. It additionally protects the frame from lung and oral hollow space cancers. Likewise, it aids the body to combat in the direction of prostate most cancers. The fruit is likewise an first-rate immune-booster. The affiliation of the antioxidant nutrients (Vitamins C, A, and E) collectively with specific anti-developing antique nutrients make the fruit a fantastic anti-ageing food deliver.

Guava offers resistance toward contamination and resistance in opposition to cancer. It furthermore continues healthful blood vessels due to the antioxidants, B-complicated, magnesium, and other comparable functioning nutrients loaded in the fruit. Guava furthermore purifies pores and pores and skin and body organs. It prevents wrinkles and pores and skin damage. It strengthens the bones through its Manganese,Magnesium, and Potassium. It additionally gives healthy mucus and cell membranes due to the Phosphorus substance contained in it. Guava additionally controls coronary heart rate and blood stress with the help of potassium and magnesium materials.

The fruit is incredible for giving notable greatest fitness and to suppose that the fruit may be very reasonably-priced and taken into consideration a completely not unusual outside and farm fruit in international locations that typically domesticate it.

Picking and Storage

The guava fruit voluntarily falls off the tree whilst it's far ripe but it is able to additionally be harvested manually. One need to be cautious in deciding on guavas due to the fact the fruit stops ripening as soon as it's miles plucked from the tree. Yellow or shiny green is a sign of ripeness in guavas. In choosing the fruit, choose ripe guavas to be plucked.If it releases without issues from the stem, it is prepared for harvest. A picker want to taste to test one of the harvested quit end result for ripeness. Some kind of guavas has white flesh however is already ripe.

Guavas can be saved in a properly-ventilated room for as lots as five weeks. However, ripe guavas can be saved in a fridge

APPLE
(Malus Domestica)
The apple is a member of the pear circle of relatives. This fruit varies in colour, taste, and texture. There are purple, inexperienced, and yellow apples. The indoors flesh is juicy and crunchy white, with small dark brown seeds at the

middle of the fruit. Apple is local to Europe and Western Asia.

Nutrients in Apple

Most of the apple's vitamins are placed on its pores and pores and pores and skin and under. It is known for its great source of pectin and fibers. The nutritional profile of 1 cup of apple (quartered or chopped) this is about a hundred twenty five grams is displayed on this desk.

Note:If a specific nutrient isn't always present, it does now not generally recommend that the fruit has none of it. It approach that the nutrient's amount of recognition does not meet the rating tool standards.

Benefits of Apple

Eating an apple ordinary is a tremendous turning factor for the body's healthful weight-reduction plan as the fruit includes phytonutrients and awesome health boosters desired in preserving the body's accurate shape. Apple enables keep away from the danger of bronchial bronchial asthma assaults thru its Vitamin C. Eating apple gets rid of frame pressure because of strenuous works. This is because of the polyphenols present within the fruit. The regular intake of this fruit reduces oxidative harm in the body that is due to free radicals. From oxidative strain bureaucracy atherosclerosis or clogged arteries. Including apples in someone's day by day eating regimen prevents or reduces the risks of atherosclerosis.

The consumption of apples moreover prevents osteoporosis due to its Calcium, Magnesium, and Manganese. It is proper for the diet of the aged. It moreover keeps wholesome gums and cavity-free tooth. As it's far protected in the regular food regimen, the fruit helps decrease the danger of diabetes because of its fiber content material fabric. Likewise, a healthy bowel motion is also ensured with apples' fiber. This approach a decrease chance of obtaining colon maximum cancers and one-of-a-kind digestive tract infections.

Apples help ease or save you fibromyalgia. The stability of Potassium and Calcium within the apple is an advantage for this shape of muscle sickness. The fruit additionally consists of Vitamin E this is some other nutrient that lets in prevent fibromyalgia. Apples also are accurate for the food regimen of these vulnerable to lung most cancers. Vitamin E permits in preventing this dangerous ailment, on the factor of various beneficial nutrients contained in apple.

Picking and Storage

Apples are available complete twelve months round in particular in shops. In picking apples, it's far first rate to pick out

out the ones who have vibrant and rich shades with a reddish red tinge at the pores and skin. A picker can climb the apple tree for higher goals or selections. Just lessen the stem from the department or twist and pluck it. Do not pull the apple off its stem because it will leave a wound at the fruit's pores and pores and skin which can cause rot in a few unspecified time in the future of storage. Avoid apples with heavy marks at the pores and skin's ground.

Apples are saved in humid locations which can be free from unwanted smells due to the reality the fruit with out troubles absorbs smells from its environment. One can also keep the harvested apples in a fridge for each different three weeks especially if the give up result are to be used for extraordinary uses or processing. However, washing the give up give up end result have to now not be neglected a good way to remove dangerous dirt and pesticide remnants.

APRICOT

## (Prunus Armeniaca)

Apricots are rounded, small orange-coloured forestall result that originated, and have been first cultivated in China. It is a member of the Rosaceae own family, collectively with peach, plum, apple, and pear. Its medical name is Prunus Armeniaca. The fruit is tart-flavored with a velvety texture.

Nutrients in Apricot

The fruit typically consists of Vitamin A, Vitamin C, Beta-Carotene, Zeaxanthin, Iron, Lycopene (as anti-oxidant), Potassium, Fiber, Pantothenic acid, and Pyridoxine. These had been considered to be placed in a small apricot fruit, which offer beneficial vitamins to the frame. Unlike extraordinary culmination, apricot is not too famous. However, its richness with a number of the critical nutrients made it a often going on and sought-after disorder-combating crop.

Below is a chart describing the vitamins located in apricot.
Benefits of Apricot

Not most effective does apricot deliver delectable taste as it's miles eaten, it moreover offers suitable fitness benefits to the handiest who consumes it. Raw or dried, the fruit extends sustenance no longer simply interior however additionally out of doors the physical body.

As a rich deliver of Vitamin A, it offers proper eyesight and pores and skin nourishment. It is even used as body and facial scrub to make pores and pores and skin feel and look more younger. The Vitamin C in apricot also boosts the frame's immune device relative to not unusual colds and one-of-a-kind infections. It has the capability to short repair wounds, lessen hypertension, and combat eye troubles together with cataracts.

Beta carotene as anti-oxidant fights the improvement of vintage-elderly diseases like arthritis and prostate most cancers in guys. Other cancers also can be prevented, similarly to coronary coronary heart ailments and the formation of stroke. Lycopene performs the same as Beta carotene in preventing cancer and bone-associated ailments, but is taken into consideration a higher anti-oxidant than the alternative. Potassium is likely to lessen the dangers of coronary coronary heart disorder and most cancers, too. Zeaxanthin, as an alternative, is every an anti-oxidant and an anti inflammatory phytochemical nutrient this is taken into consideration as a first-rate nutrient for the eye. Being nicely nourished with it method having a healthful and younger searching eye.

Another essential mineral decided in apricot is Iron. It is an energy booster with the primary characteristic of sporting oxygen from the lungs to the muscle groups and exclusive frame organs. Lack of this nutrient consequences to having anemia, and if untreated, may additionally bring about distinct extreme headaches. Pantothenic acidhelps enhance the body's strength and metabolism, combat stress and nasal infections, heal wounds, and prevent zits from coming once more. While Pyridoxine as each other apricot advantage, efficaciously treats menstrual issues, heart, and kidney ailments.

Picking and Storage

Like different quit result, apricots aren't allowed to ripen on the tree. It have to be picked at the identical time as still agency but with a bit softness to it. The shade must be deep yellow or orange with a trace of crimson on its ground. Do no longer choose out individuals who despite the fact that have sun shades of inexperienced to ripen them similarly on the tree. Unripe apricots are first rate stored in a refrigerator inner a plastic bag at room temperature. Leave the end result there for up to three days. Ripe ones may be positioned in plastic food savers and saved in a fridge for every extraordinary 3 to 4 days.

## BANANA

Banana is a protracted, curved fruit that grows in clusters with candy tasting gentle flesh. It is taken into consideration as one of the earliest cultivated give up result from the circle of relatives Musaceae. Its name is taken from an Arab phrase "Banan," which means finger. It is an ageless plant with long and massive palm-like leaves. The banana tree bears male and lady plant life at the age of maturity, but great the girl blossom turns into culmination. The bunch of overturned stop stop end result seems like "palms," at the same time as each banana is referred to as "finger."

Nutrients in Banana

A medium-sized banana gives sufficient quantity of anti-oxidants, nutrients, and minerals. It has accurate results at the fitness of folks who frequently eat it. The fruit is considered as one of the healthiest vegetation determined in the marketplace this is proper for a person's every day food plan.

Below is a table of crucial vitamins determined in a medium-sized banana.
Note:If a selected nutrient isn't gift, it does no longer generally advise that the fruit has none of it. It method that the nutrient's quantity of recognition does now not meet the score device standards.

Health Benefits

Banana is one of the maximum nutritious fruits within the global. It incorporates 3 natural sugars mainly: sucrose, glucose, and fructose. If those sugars are combined with fiber which is also observed in banana, our frame could have widespread amount of power. This is why banana is so famous with athletes. Two bananas an afternoon offer them sufficient deliver of power for sporting activities.

Banana lets in lessen despair with its Potassium plus Vitamins A and C which reinforces and strengthens the mind. It moreover boosts mind energy by way of giving an alert thoughts. The deliciously sweet fruit also prevents anemia. Bananas are immoderate in Iron, a nutrient that fights this sort of disorder. The fiber in banana stops constipation and diarrhea and it normalizes bowel functions. If wholesome bones are what a person goals, the fruit is a good benefit as it strengthens bones through its Calcium.

Banana additionally includes antioxidant vitamins that reduce the risk of kidney most cancers, and its immoderate Potassium content material fabric makes it a relevant fruit for hypertensive sufferers.

The fruit has natural antacid that is a awesome treatment for heartburn. It additionally improves blood-sugar levels specifically the "Banaba," a kind of banana that enables cope with diabetes. With the fruit's fiber income the benefit of decreasing acidity within the stomach as it is an powerful treatment for gastritis and ulcers. Banana is likewise an top notch protector of eyesight due to its antioxidants in particular the Vitamin C. The fruit furthermore lets in relieve pressure by using manner of controlling heartbeat and the body's water balance with it Potassium. The Vitamin B6in banana also aids in enhancing nerve competencies. Ultimately, banana has cooling results at the body and is called the "cooling fruit" as it permits manage frame temperature.

Picking and Storage

Ripe bananas have wealthy perfume, are pretty organization, and bright yellow in coloration. The pores and skin is easy to peel and the fruit tastes candy. Bananas are typically harvested on the same time as although green. Nevertheless, the harvester has the discretion to pick out the fruit or permit it stay on its tree, depending on his intake eagerness or exceptional plans. Because bananas are fragile, safety against grazes ought to be taken into consideration throughout garage period. Bananas need to be saved in a room temperature so as to finish ripening method. Storing unripe bananas in a fridge is unwise as it will interrupt its ripening approach. To quicken banana ripening, truely located the fruit in a plastic or paper wrap.

Bananas can be stored in a freezer if bear in mind to be consumed at a later time. Sprinkling it with lemon juice prevents discoloration till the fruit is ready to apply.

## BLUEBERRIES

Blueberries are the size of grapes; small and rounded blue violet end give up result from the heath circle of relatives Ericaceae. These originated from North America mainly in Minnesota. The fruit is a favourite of the Native Americans. Usually planted on acid soil, the shrubs of those little flowers inside the suggest time are developed within the East and West.

Nutrients in Blueberries

Blueberries rank highest in illness-preventing antioxidants. Among extraordinary wholesome surrender result, blueberries had been considered because the "Super Food." The benefit of this fruit inside the healthy dietweight-reduction plan is diagnosed with the useful resource of fitness agencies, and the American Cancer Society located blueberry at the top of its list of ingredients useful in competition to superb sorts of cancers. This chart enumerated the dietary portions of blueberries in line with 1 cup (approx. 148g).

Health Benefits

Though blueberries do no longer taste like one-of-a-type pungently candy end end result, the ones small attractively colored flowers contain hundreds of nutrients. The fruit has fitness-selling phytochemical related to antioxidant and anti-growing older advantages. It moreover promotes healthful urinary tract with out infections via its antibiotic homes that help cleanse bacteria building up inside the tract. Blueberry's characteristic in enhancing night time imaginative and prescient and popular eye care is that it carries antioxidants blended with Vitamin C, A&E, Zinc, Selenium, and Phosphorus. This is why the fruit is so appropriate for the eye.

The antioxidants in blueberry which includes proanthocyanidins, resveratrol, flavonols, and tannins assist prevent increase of most cancers cells in particular colon and ovarian cancers. The immoderate cognizance of antioxidants inside the fruit earned it the decision, "the antioxidant first-rate fruit." Likewise, the antioxidants furthermore promote anti-growing older and guard towards continual heartdiseases. This is thru neutralizing the radicals in order to maintain it at bay.

Blueberries moreover save you the infection of Alzheimer's illness andbrain getting older. It has herbal mind food that reverses reminiscence loss and permits with motor competencies and the assist of the antioxidant, Vitamin C. The Copper and acids found in blueberry useful resource in enhancing from diarrhea and decorate the frame's digestion. The nutrients C, B complex, E&A, Iron, Zinc, and Copperboost up the immune gadget. Copper is a very effective anti-bacterial and immune builder. This lets in lessen the replication of HIV.

Blueberry is considerable in Vitamin C combined with anthocyanidins, which strengthen the body's collagen. Collagen is an crucial bond making the pores and skin, gums, and joint bendy however strong.Blueberry is also an anti-diabetes meals due to its abundance in antioxidants and Potassium. In evaluating blueberries to nearly forty healthful stop cease end result and veggies, it were given the very high-quality score on the subject of the above-stated fitness advantages.

Picking and Storage

A better manner to choose blueberries is to find out a terrific bush with a bucket tied to your waist. Ripe genuine ones are blue and the skins are not crazed. The larger berry, the sweeter it's miles. In order to pick out a couple of berries unto your bucket, attempt cupping the bunch associated with the stem and lightly rub it. Ripe berries will resultseasily fall into your fingers because of the truth the more youthful ones remain related to the bush. Be careful in selecting blueberries as they're able to stain palms and clothes. Also, if you are selecting within the wilds, be with distinct humans. The fruit is likewise well-known with unique wild animals like undergo. This animal loves blueberry.

After selecting, dispose of imperfect berries from the best ones. Put them in glass or plastic boxes as metals purpose discoloration. Leave the bins open on the manner to prevent moisture that still impacts the coloration of the berries. Do not wash the berries if now not to be consumed or used proper away as this will cause them to soggy. If the berries are to be frozen, located them in freezer bins with out washing to keep its herbal texture. But consider to clean the berries in cold water in advance than using.

CANTALOUPE
(Cucumis Melo)

Cantaloupes are rounded, candy fragrant fruit with soft juicy flesh of pinkish-orange whilst ripe. Cantaloupe is likewise referred to as Muskmelon, which is thought to be first cultivated in Egypt and Greece because of its portrayal in Egyptian art work in the course of Biblical period. Others believed that it originated from Persia, India, or Africa. However, its proper basis is inconclusive as much as the cutting-edge. The fruit is a member of the gourd family Cucurbitaceae. The clinical call of cantaloupe is Cucumis Melo with seven unique botanical versions.

## Nutrients in Cantaloupe

Cantaloupe is a delight to weight-losers. It has zero fats and honestly low in calories. It has Vitamin A gain over a few healthy fruits and vegetables. Approximately one-fourth of a medium-sized cantaloupe is stated to be with 4450 IU.

Confirming the important nutrients placed in a glowing, one hundred grams cantaloupe is a nutrients table given under.

## Benefits of Cantaloupe

Cantaloupe is rich in fitness-promoting nutrients required for extremely good physical condition. These lists of health advantages are dominant within the fruit. Cantaloupe is a absolutely fat-free meals. Diets which might be low in common fat prevent the improvement of cancers; even as diets low in saturated fats lessen the threat of coronary coronary coronary heart sicknesses.The fruit is likewise very low in sodium. It lowers blood stress as a quit result averting hypertensive attacks in someone.

The fruit serves as diureticbecause it is considerable in Potassium, and having excessive water content material could be very useful to excessive blood strain sufferers. The risk of having a infant with mind and spinal twine defects is averted because of the folic acid located in cantaloupe.Good eyesight and pores and pores and skin are also a outstanding benefit that the fruit gives. It has very excessive Vitamin A and Cthat promotes specific imaginative and prescient and wholesome sparkling pores and pores and skin unfastened from infections and viruses. Cantaloupe is likewise wealthy in antioxidant such Lutein that offers eye health.

Cantaloupe is a fantastic anti-growing old meals as it gives power and flexibility to the skin, gums, and joints. High amount of Vitamin Cbuilds frame tissues healthily for a extra younger physical glow. It additionally enables smooth phlegm and relieves tuberculosis coughwith its Vitamin Athat promotes lung health. A deficiency with the perfect nutrients results in lung ailments and emphysema and the extremely good manner to keep away from these is to embody the vitamin within the every day healthy dietweight-reduction plan. Eating cantaloupe additionally relaxes toothachebecause of the Vitamin A and Calciumthat sell sturdy bones and enamel.

Other advantages from cantaloupe are healthful urinary tract, smooth intestines, cushty temperament, mouth rinse, and it furthermore cools fever.

Picking and Storage

Heavy cantaloupes are more likely to be ripe and the rinds are clean. Ready to pick out out out ripe cantaloupes have layers of colour and they're neither colourful nor stupid in texture. There ought to be a tinge of yellow and a grayish tan for it to be picked. Ripe ones have sturdy aromatic perfume so it is not difficult to determine it from the immature ones. Plus, ripe cantaloupes are softly employer however now not overly. Hard ones are genuinely unripe. Avoid cantaloupes which may be bruised and grazed.

For exquisite garage, vicinity the fruit in a fab ventilated place at home. Those with reduce sections have to be placed in a fridge. Wash cantaloupes and decrease in halves to discard the seeds and strings using a spoon. Cut in desired sizes.

CRANBERRIES

(Vaccinium Macrocarpon)

Cranberry is a fruit of small creeping flowers, usually a vine of the family Ericaceae that is related to cranberries. The clinical call of the fruit is Vaccinium Macrocarpon with 4 certainly one of a kind versions. The Native Americans in North America have been the number one to use cranberries as meals. Besides North America, the fruit is likewise placed in marshy lands of Asia, Northern and Central Europe. Cranberries ripen in September and feature bitter flavor that overpowers its sweetness.

Nutrients in Cranberries

Cranberries or bounceberries aren't very well-known like superb berries. But there are extra health advantages within the fruit than with the others which might be placed in market. Another suitable detail is that it's miles a great deal much less highly-priced but with greater of the health-promoting benefits for the body.

This chart shows the in-intensity predominant nutrients in 1 cup of cranberries.

Note:If a particular nutrient isn't present, it does now not commonly endorse that the fruit has none of it. It approach that the nutrient's amount of cognizance does not meet the score device necessities.

Benefits of Cranberries

Cranberries have majority of phytonutrients aside from its foremost vitamins like Vitamin C, fiber, and Manganese. These unique vitamins encompass antioxidant, anti-inflammatory, and anti-maximum cancers homes. Speaking of the fruit's health advantages, the most usually believed cranberry juice extracted from its berries absolutely lacks the overall phytonutrients blessings coming from it. The "whole fruit" have to be fed on because it has the entire bulk of the array of phytonutrients.

Cranberries shield in competition to urinary tract infection. The culmination functionality to offer healthful urinary tract is credited to its Proanthocyanidins, this is a sort of phytonutrient. It stops fine types of bacteria to go into the urinary tract linings. The fruit also acts as anti-inflammatory. Cranberries shield the frame toward undesirable infection of the gums, colon, and the blood vessels.

The intake of cranberries reduces the improvement of kidney stones – no matter the truth that there are studies that relate the intake of cranberry to the formation of kidney stones, the urinary uric acid is decreased by way of the consumption of cranberries due to this the danger of kidney stones to willing people is likewise lessened. However, it is probably best to are seeking for recommendation from a health care expert upon the inclusion of cranberry on their weight loss plan.

The fruit additionally lets in the immune device as it lessens the flu and bloodless infection on the frame through its antioxidant Vitamin C. A wholesome aerobic-vascular device is also a gain that comes from consuming the fruit. Its antioxidants play a vital function in maintaining healthy blood vessels associated with high blood pressure and exceptional cardio-vascular illnesses. Theantioxidants in cranberries offer us with the strongest fitness benefits.

Cranberries are a wealthy supply of flavonoid quercetin that could hold once more the development of breast and colon cancers. This is why the fruit is an anti-most cancers food.

Picking and Storage

High-first-rate cranberries are business business enterprise to touch with the shade of pink. Firmness is a primary signal of having tremendous fine. Picking calls for no precise handling as those matured quit end result are robust. Sorting right cranberries from the lesser ones makes use of the bouncing technique. Good extremely good berries soar better than the others and as a end end result picked and separated.

There are fast strategies of harvesting cranberries however hand-deciding on this is usually used is the most secure way simply so the vines will have lesser harm.

Ripe and clean cranberries can be stored in a refrigerator for 20 days. However, shrunk or faulty ones need to be discarded so you can avoid contaminating the superb ones. Damp berries sparkling from the refrigerator aren't spoiled. Signs of spoilage are discoloration and stickiness. Frozen cranberries can be saved in a freezer for numerous years the use of a freezer bag. Once the fruits are defrosted, they want to be used or consumed proper now.

FIG

Figs are deliciously candy combined with a chewy clean flesh. The seeds of this fruit are crunchy, too. The Ficus tree (Ficus carica L.) from the Mulberry circle of relatives grows the figs. The fruit develops with the help of the surroundings thru an opening referred to as "ostiole" or "eye." Figs are believed to be a community to West Asia and later allocated to the Mediterranean.

Nutrients in Fig

Figs are luscious and nutritious seasonal give up end result. This fruit varies in coloration and texture. Majority of figs are dried through publicity within the warm temperature of the solar or artificial techniques. The chart under offers

151

information of the number one nutrient placed in figs.

Value of nutrients consistent with 1 massive fig (approx. Sixty four g):

Note:If a particular nutrient isn't always present, it does no longer typically mean that the fruit has none of it. It approach that the nutrient's amount of focus does now not meet the rating system necessities.

Benefits of Figs

Health blessings of figs are attributed to the principle vitamins, minerals, and fiber which might be located inside the fruit. Figs sell low cholesterol. Fibercontent of the fruit washes out ldl ldl cholesterol in the digestive tool and out of body. It stops coronary coronary heart diseasewith the Omega-6 fatty acids decided in it which lessens the hazard of coronary coronary heart illnesses.

The fruit prevents colon and breast cancers. This is with the assist of its fiber content. The nutrient furthermore enables in having healthful bowels, so figs are beneficial in preventing constipation. Figs additionally assist lessen weight but if fed on with milk, weight gain is the quit end result. The fruit is also applicable for diabetesas it Potassium enables manage blood sugar and fig leaves have anti-diabetic residences. Figs are excessive in Potassium but low in Sodium. If blanketed within the weight-reduction plan, it is able to reduce the threat of excessive blood strain. However, an excessive amount of intake of figs reasons diarrhea.

Eating figs inside the morning improves sexual power. It improves sexual powers. The fruit additionally promotes hard bones due to its Calcium which strengthens the bones. The one-of-a-kind blessings of the fruit are throat comfort and specific eyesight

Picking and Storage

Ready to reap figs have candy perfume due to the fact sour odor manner spoilage. Pick figs which is probably plum and clean with deep coloring. They ought to be bruise-free and feature enterprise company stems.

Ripe figs need to be in a refrigerator for up to 2 days. Figs are sensitive absolutely in order that they want to be wrapped in paper towels or plastic boxes in order now not to bruise or lure smell from close by ingredients. If figs are unripe, they need to be positioned in a plate and stored at a room temperature without daylight. Similarly, dried figs need to be saved in a refrigerator and nicely-wrapped in order that they may not be exposed to cold air a great way to cause hardness.

GRAPEFRUIT
(Citrus paradisi)

Grapefruit (Citrus paradisi) is a favourite citrus fruit loved via many human beings spherical the arena. It is eaten as breakfast or perhaps snacks. The fruit's juicy sweetness competes with that of the oranges, and it secures a excessive place among many citrus culmination. The fruit is said to originate from the island of Barbados and taken to Jamaica, ordinary with facts.

Nutrients in Grapefruit

The health advantages of grapefruit are widespread and without same. It is an fantastic supply of Vitamin C like different citrus end end result. Grapefruit is idea to be a effective drug-poison eliminator.

Examining the chart below will tell you of all the principle vitamins decided in a 1 cup of grapefruit, (approx. 230 g).

Note:If a specific nutrient isn't always gift, it does no longer necessarily endorse that the fruit has none of it. It manner that the nutrient's quantity of awareness does now not meet the rating tool requirements.

Health Benefits of Grapefruit

Because of its health-selling vitamins, grapefruit have become named the "fruit of paradise." It is loaded with Vitamin C like terrific citrus culmination. The fruit has immoderate water content material material fabric and much a whole lot less sodium. It is likewise immoderate in enzymes. With these three present characteristics, the body's metabolism will increase. Meaning, grapefruit allows in losing weight.

Grapefruit strengthens the immune gadget. The Vitamin C reduces cold symptoms and symptoms, arthritis, bronchial asthma, rheumatism, cancers, strokes, and fortifies cardiovascular fitness stopping the hazard of coronary coronary heart attacks.Also, the Lycopene in grapefruit permits fight prostate cancer, and tumors.

Grapefruit additionally permits combat colon most cancers, lung and oral cavity cancers, and protects pores and pores and skin from UV rays.

Picking and Storage

The season of grapefruit is from September to December. In choosing it, keep away from people who have wrinkled and overly difficult texture of skin as the ones are thick-skinned grapefruits. The fruit must be corporation however barely gentle. Keep at room temperature.

Before consumption, wash grapefruits in cool water so as now not to switch micro organism into the fruit's flesh as quickly because it has been reduce. It may be chilled however the perfume is not as robust as those saved in a room.

GRAPES

Grapes are translucent, clean-skinned spherical berries that broaden in clusters from woody vines of genus Vitis. These fruits both have appropriate for ingesting seeds or seedless. Grapes are community to the a few areas of Mediterranean and Europe and is now in massive thing cultivated spherical the sector.

Nutrients in Grapes

Grapes are taken into consideration one of the most favored end end result inside the global. Aside from this, it includes loads of useful fitness nutrients which can be suitable for the body. Some of the principle vitamins in grapes are the following:

This rating have emerge as taken from 1 cup grapes (approx. 151 g).

Note:If a specific nutrient isn't always present, it does no longer constantly mean that the fruit has none of it. It method that the nutrient's quantity of hobby does not meet the score machine standards.

Health Benefits of Grapes

Deliciously juicy grapes make sure healthy and active lifestyles. Many fitness blessings are discovered inside the fruit containing flavonoids which can be effective antioxidants to useful resource the body in in competition to developing older. Grapes save you coronary coronary heart illnesses because of its antioxidant this is the Vitamin C. The culmination help in preventing blood clots inflicting heart attacks. This is as it will boom nitric oxide stages inside the blood. Grapes additionally address migraine. It must be consumed early in the morning as home remedy for migraine. It want to now not be blended with water. The antioxidants in grapes enhance the body's power due to this, providing immediately energy and fights fatigue. Likewise, the fruit remedy alternatives indigestion inside the stomach and forestalls dyspepsia via its fiber content fabric.

Eating the fruit reduces the improvement of mammary tumor due to its crimson colored Concord, preventing breast most cancers. The fruit is taken into consideration as laxative due to containing herbal acid, sugar, and cellulose. Thus, it lessens constipation. A phytonutrient named resveratrol is observed to be placed in grape seeds and flesh. It lets in the body have durability and anti-developing older advantages. This phytonutrient also complements mind health and lessens the tiers of amyloidal-beta peptides in patients with Alzheimer's disease.

Flavonoids as antioxidant are positioned in grapes that fight the harm because of unfastened radicals. It additionally stops cataract formation inside the eyes. Grapes are anti-bacterial forestall give up end result and that they help save you infections. For the bronchial bronchial asthma patients, the fruit is high first rate because it can help remedy hypersensitive reactions and increase the moisture in lungs due to the presence of the Vitamin C in it.

Picking and Storage

Grapes are available inside the direction of every season. Ripened grapes need to have a pinkish pink tinge at the same time as green ones have to have yellowish tinge. Fully ripened grapes are fleshy and easy, and are unfastened from crinkles. The end end result are effects spoiled so they need to be saved in a refrigerator inner a plastic bag or airtight packing containers.

KIWI FRUIT

(Actinidia deliciosa)

Kiwi (Actinidia deliciosa) is an oval-formed fruit with mild brown pores and skin that has exquisite tiny hairs. Inside is an emerald inexperienced flesh that embraces small black seeds. The center or center of the fruit is a white flesh. This has numerous tastes collectively with sweet, tart, and at instances acidic. All the components of the fruit is said to be steady to devour. The fruit is likewise taken into consideration as natural because its tree is alternatively evidence towards parasites, which frees it from pesticides and special dangerous organisation substance. Kiwi is nearby to China with the precise name of Yang Tao. However, after being introduced to New Zealand through missionaries, the choice modified into changed after the population of the location known as "Kiwi." The fruit is China's country wide fruit.

Nutrients in Kiwi

Kiwi fruit is complete of healthy vitamins. The fruit is thought for its Vitamin C content material material which has more quantity than orange. It is likewise a amazing supply of nutritional fiber. Below is a chart containing the number one vitamins in 1 cup of Kiwi, it honestly is about 177 grams.

Note:If a selected nutrient isn't gift, it does not always recommend that the fruit has none of it. It manner that the nutrient's amount of cognizance does now not meet the score system necessities.

Health Benefits of Kiwi Fruit

The vitamins and minerals in Kiwi fruit makes it useful for notable illnesses and conditions. The fruit additionally consists of phytonutrients that sell health. Eating Kiwi fruit is a wholesome preference and it is particularly beneficial with bronchial allergic reactions as it prevents coughing and wheezing in particular in kids. The immoderate tiers of Vitamin C in the fruit work advantageously in this example. Kiwi fruit additionally keeps the frame's deoxyribonucleic acid from mutations, because of this it protects the DNA.

Kiwi consists of excellent quantities of Vitamin C, E and A tested to protect our frame in the direction of unfastened radicals and ailments which include hypertension, weight issues, and most cancers particularly in the colon. The fruit moreover improves the safety closer to diabetesthrough it fiber content material that controls the quantity of sugar in the body. It is a exceptional gain to have easy eyes and kiwi reduces the chance of eye-associated illnesses through the use of 36% and forestalls vision impairment. This is with the assist of Vitamin C within the fruit.

The aggregate of Calcium, Magnesium, and Vitamin Eprevents cramping of muscle tissues within the frame. Magnesium is a top notch bone-strengthening mineral like Calcium. Also, kiwi's vitamins restriction neuronal harm in the brain, therefore preventing Alzheimer's disorder inside the aged. The fruit is likewise beneficial for pregnant ladies because of the truth the Folate in it's far an adequate and suitable vitamins for the development of an unborn little one's mind and spinal twine. Likewise, Folate consumption lessens despair in addition to dementia. Adequate Folate degrees are also critical for proper mind functioning. It slows down the effects of getting older.

Picking and Storage

Kiwi end end result are available for the duration of maximum of the one year. However, the fruit is at its best all through August to November. It is straightforward to pick Kiwi fruit due to the fact while you hold it amongst your thumb and forefingers and look at mild stress, it's going to yield right now. Those that don't yield aren't ripe but. Very gentle kiwis with damp spots need to be prevented.

However, the fruit can be left to ripen for up to six days. Put it in plastic bag collectively with an apple or a banana that permits you to hasten its ripeness.

LEMON/LIME

Lemons(Citrus Limon) are oval and yellow citrus stop end result with coarse outer pores and pores and skin. The common lemon has 8 to ten segments of refreshingly juicy, tart and acidic internal flesh. Lemons are clearly bitter but there are also candy types which is probably well-known in consuming places and markets.

Limes(Citrus Aurantifolia) but, are a small citrus fruit which can be green in pores and pores and skin and flesh. It can be spherical or oval with a diameter that stages among 1 to two inches. The fruit also may be bitter or candy.

Nutrient in Lemon/Lime

Lemons and limes are notable assets of Vitamin C. These are the maximum extensively used citrus fruits inside the global and encompass more health reaping blessings vitamins than oranges and the others.

The chart under describes the vitamins in keeping with 1 fruit without a seed (approx. 108 g).

Note: If a specific nutrient is not present, it does no longer necessarily advocate that the fruit has none of it. It way that the nutrient's quantity of awareness does no longer meet the rating tool necessities.

Health Benefits of Lemon/Lime Citrus cease stop end result are valued for his or her nutritious and antioxidant homes. They have many tested fitness benefits together with preventing scurvy. This disorder is due to a deficiency in Vitamin C that is characterised with the aid of cough and colds, cracked lips and lip corners, swollen and bleeding gums, and ulcers in tongue. The remedy is having sufficient quantity of Vitamin C within the frame. Lemons and limes are blessed with this and they prevent scurvy if blanketed inside the eating regimen.

Lemon and lime rejuvenates the pores and pores and skin while taken orally or executed. They moreover lessen frame fragrance. The acids in lemon or lime scrub away useless pores and pores and skin cells whilst rubbed anywhere inside the body. The stop result have whitening agent and are extensively used as pores and pores and skin whiteners especially inside the underarms. They smoothen and whiten pores and skin. The give up end result' acids stimulate the digestive device, growing the secretion of digestive juices and gives wholesome digestion to those who encompass the prevent result on their food regimen.

The give up give up result are also used as decongestant. It offers treatment from congestion and nausea. It aids in promoting respiratory fitness. This is due to the Flavonoids within the stop stop result. For folks that are trimming their body down, the citric acid located within the culmination is a first rate fats burner. Thus, the prevent end end result are essential for weight reduction. For eye care, the antioxidants in Vitamin Cprotect the eyes from developing older and macular degeneration.

Lemon and lime are also appropriate appetizers, treatments arthritis, rheumatism, prostrate and colon cancers, cholera, arteriosclerosis, diabetes, fatigue, coronary heart illnesses or maybe very excessive fever (in opposite to famous belief). These are the alternative blessings a person could have via the consumption of those healthy citrus end end result.

Picking and Storage

Lemons are available all yr spherical. Full yellow colour is an indication that a lemon is already ripe. Choose skinny-skinned and heavy ones for choosing as the ones show whole ripeness. Having a tinge of green within the fruit way it is not absolutely ripe. Likewise,in deciding on limes, pick out out out those which might be heavy and huge for his or her size. Skin should be deep inexperienced in shade. Limes flip yellow as they ripen but the top of their tartness is when they are even though green. Avoid limes that have brownish tinge as their flavors are quiterotten.

Lemons and limes ought to be saved at room temperature far from direct sunlight hours. Exposure to sun turns those end result into yellow and affects their herbal flavors. If stored well, the ones stop end result will live smooth for a week. They also can be refrigerated in a plastic bag and placed within the refrigerator crisper to keep freshness for up to fourteen days. Juices of lemon and lime additionally can be stored inside the fridge for later use.

ORANGES
(Citrus Sinensis)

The orange fruit is round-fashioned with leathery and porous pores and pores and pores and skin. The colour is from orange to crimson orange. It is one of the commonplace grown end result within the international. Other kinds of oranges make up about -thirds of all oranges which can be grown international. Oranges is stated to have originated in Southeast Asia and later cultivated in China in 2500 BC.

Nutrients in Oranges

It is scientifically set up that oranges have many showed health advantages. The fruit carries many quantities of vitamins and minerals. As you examine the chart beneath, you may see the primary nutrients in oranges. The identical price of those vitamins became taken from 1 cup of oranges of about 100 seventy grams.

Note:If a specific nutrient isn't gift, it does now not constantly advise that the fruit has none of it. It manner that the nutrient's amount of attention does no longer meet the score tool standards.

Health Benefits of Oranges

Oranges have greater flavonoids and phytonutrients and are established to have anti-tumor, anti-inflammatory, and antioxidant homes.

The fiber in oranges stimulates digestive juices therefore relieving constipation. Consumption of oranges makes someone avoid kidney ailments because of the truth eating orange juice reduces the danger of the formation of calcium oxalate stone in the kidney. Eating oranges moreover strengthens enamel and bonesbecause the calcium in oranges toughens the bones. Oranges moreover helps preserve healthful pores and pores and skin. The beta-carotene protects the cells from harm. It frees it from free radicals and anti-growing old.Iron and Vitamin B6aid in the production of hemoglobin consequently, purifying the blood. Oranges protects the blood from viral infections.

The fruit is also an anti-most cancers agent. The immoderate amount of Vitamin C in oranges prevents cellular damage and placed away unfastened radicals. It prevents lung, oral, colon, and breast cancers. The fruit is right for hypertensive men and women because it lowers high blood stress. The Magnesium in oranges continues the blood pressureand the flavonoids alter it.

Picking and Storage

Choose natural oranges if possible due to the reality the fruit is some of the list of fruits that pesticide residues are in modern-day found. However, inorganic or natural the orange may be, its taste remains the identical. Avoid oranges with easy spots and mold. Choose clean skinned and heavy oranges for those have more juices.

Store at room temperature or in a fridge. Oranges are higher stored openly and now not inner plastic bins

PAPAYA
(Carica Papaya L.)

Papaya is a tropical fruit. It is from the gender Carica. It grows from a tall, woody and big herb. It might be very well-known specially for its deliciously candy taste. The fruit's pulp is deep orange that is gentle and candy. Papayas are generally served as cakes. However, shakes are a favorite for this fruit, too. There are many techniques to consume papaya. In unique worldwide locations, the fruit is cooked with coconut milk at the same time as it's far however raw. The seeds are stable to consume in spite of the truth that a bit bitter. Papayas encompass Papain, an enzyme that aids in digesting proteins in the body. Papaya is local to South Mexico and its neighboring global locations.

Nutrients in Papaya

Papaya is a incredible supply of Vitamins A and C, inclusive of various main nutrients located within the table below.

Note:If a specific nutrient is not gift, it does not always mean that the fruit has none of it. It method that the nutrient's amount of awareness does no longer meet the score tool standards.

Health Benefits of Papaya

The richness of papaya fruit in nutrients and minerals, antioxidants, and nutritional fiber makes it a nutritious food. It is even taken into consideration as one of the Super Foods. Aside from its delectably milky taste, it's far famous because of the vitamins it gives to the body. More health blessings also are given by using using way of the fruit which incorporates assisting with suitable digestion. This is due to the enzyme Papain that is decided inside the fruit. Papaya also allows deal with slipped spinal disc and pinched nerves because of its Chymopapain that is robust in treating this ailment.

Papaya reduces rheumatoid and osteoarthritis. The immoderate degree of

Vitamin C in the fruit is the best liable for this fitness advantage. The fruit moreover lowers ldl cholesterol due to its immoderate antioxidant content thatprevents ldl cholesterol oxidation. Papaya gives sturdy immunity. It prevents recurrent colds and flu due to its high Vitamin C. Likewise, this scrumptious fruit factors correct bacteria which might be suitable for the treatment of fantastic ailments. Another fitness benefit is getting rid of parasites inside the belly. Papainaids the frame in destroying intestinal worms, consequently ensuring wholesome bowel movement. During constipation, papaya allows stimulate the bowels and treat inflammatory bowel issues.

Picking and Storage

Papaya is chosen steady with its meant use. It may be picked ripe or inexperienced. Green papayas are meant for cooking. If you want to consume ripe papaya, you may select one that has a tinge of yellowish orange and allow it ripen through garage. Papaya fruit grows from a tall tree of 10 to twelve inches or extra. You can climb up the tree or use lengthy poles with connected improvised blade at the tip to cut the stem that is related to the branch.Spots in papaya are no huge deal. It is normally determined at the papaya skins. However, keep away from those who've bruised and overly moderate due to the fact those are actually in decay.

Papayas that aren't truly ripe are saved at room temperature in case you want to ripen
Put in a plastic bag with a banana to hasten the ripening approach. If reduce, installation a refrigerator and consume inside 2 days surely so its delicious flavor might be loved.

PEARS
(Pyrus Communis)

Pears are yellow or inexperienced stop result which might be candy and juicy. This fruit is a own family of the apple. It ranks 2nd as the favorite fruit of the usa. They are rounded fruits that grow to be narrower to the stalk. Textures are smooth and barely grainy. The fruit is associated with the apple, and moreover envelopes numerous seeds at the middle. The not unusual pear fruit originated from Europe.

Nutrients in Pears

The pear is rich in fitness boosting vitamins and continues the frame in amazing shape. It is beneficial for folks who watch their weight loss plan due to it's miles low in power.

This dietary profile is taken from 1 cup of pear.

Note:If a specific nutrient is not gift, it does not usually advocate that the fruit has none of it. It manner that the nutrient's quantity of attention does not meet the score device requirements.

Health Benefits of Pears

Pears can boost the frame's electricity ranges. This fruit must be included in an individual's eating regimen as it offers lots of advantage to the body's health problems. Pears promote weight reduction. The fruit is low in calories making it nicely for individuals who watch their waistlines. It is also an electricity booster. Pear is a extraordinary supply of natural strength. Likewise, the sugar content fabric of pear permits in exercising patience.

Another fitness advantage that comes from the fruit is its ability to lower blood stress. The antioxidantsplus Potassiumhelp adjust blood pressure in particular for parents that are hypertensive. With this, a healthful cardiovascular tool is acquired. A healthy colon is every other benefit given with the useful resource of pears. Fiber binds maximum cancers-inflicting chemical materials that harm the colon cells. It moreover permits protect toward breast maximum cancers. Eating the fruit and collectively with it in a regular weight loss plan can save you most cancers cells in these regions of the frame to get up. Good eyesight makes one centered and alert and pears have this gain. It offers precise eyesight and smooth imaginative and prescient. The antioxidant (Vitamin C) gives this beneficial resource. With this vitamins, pear will become a herbal preventative fruit for hosts of ailments superior inside the frame. It is taken into consideration anti inflammatory.

Picking and Storage

Look for pears which are enterprise however not too difficult. Pick pears when they may be almost ripe. Ripe pears fall off with out problems at the equal time as pulled from the stem. These culmination can be saved at room temperature so that you can preserve its freshness. However, they need to no longer be exposed to direct daylight due to the truth the solar's warmth should have an effect on the texture and taste of pears. If you want to maintain the fruits longer, keep it in a dark place.

PINEAPPLE
(Ananas Comosus)

Pineapples are massive tropical fruit with prickly pores and pores and skin. It is right and juicy. The colour of the pores and pores and pores and skin varies from greenish yellow to reddish yellow relying on the area of cultivation. Pineapple is quite nutritious and might gain your body in lots of methods. Pineapples are to be had within the market whole year spherical. Pineapple fruit is local to South America and no longer Hawaii. Although the fruit is associated with the tropical island as it have turn out to be its principal crop.

Nutrients in Pineapple

See what makes pineapple an incredible fruit on your food plan. The nutritional profile underneath is taken from 1 cup pineapple chunks.

Note:If a selected nutrient is not present, it does no longer normally mean that the fruit has none of it. It approach that the nutrient's quantity of interest does no longer meet the score system standards.

Health Benefits of Pineapple

Pineapples are greater than really scrumptious. They can enhance life's sturdiness via their exciting health benefits. Pineapples have excessive Vitamin Cthat protects the frame closer to viruses and builds robust skin defenses in opposition to infections. It promotes healthful cells.Pineapples are also low in Sodium, Cholesterol, and Saturated fats. These developments are important for preserving blood pressure, and for having healthy cardiovascular device.

The excellent nutrients determined in pineapple are doing all your frame a remarkable wholesome issuer. Pineapples offer healthy digestive tool. The fiber in pineapple is vital for cleansing the intestines and retaining it a ways from radicals that threaten it. It replenishes digestive juices for healthy digestion.Pineapple nutrient Bromelain permits reduce swelling in infected pores and skin and hastens the recuperation of wounds and excellent skin abnormalities. It is considered an anti inflammatory nutrient. Also, to have healthful and strong bones is a notable gain over each day tough works. Pineapple gives healthy bones. Manganesehelps form lively bones and connecting tissues.

www.ingramcontent.com/pod-product-compliance
Lightning Source LLC
Chambersburg PA
CBHW062140020426
42335CB00013B/1275